International Reflections on Approaches to Mental Health Social Work

Growing out of an interest in exploring the contemporary contexts and practices related to mental health social work across the world, this book provides a range of insights into the social factors which contribute, sometimes quite significantly, to the emergence of mental health problems for individuals and even whole communities. The range and scope of mental health social work is highlighted through the different accounts of therapeutic work, advocacy, support and rehabilitation. But this collection goes further and also provides the reader with critical analyses of social work practice and social policies in certain contexts, thus inviting the reader to a more reflective consideration of the value of mental health perspectives in social work in general.

Taken as a whole, the collection suggests that social work engages with the field of mental health in diverse, creative, and very reflective ways, yet is always focused on the needs and rights of those for whom problems with mental health can be personally challenging and often disempowering.

This book was originally published as a special issue of the *Journal of Social Work Practice*.

Malcolm Golightley is Professor of Social Work at the University of Lincoln, UK, and a registered social worker with extensive mental health experience. He is the editor of the *British Journal of Social Work*.

Gloria Kirwan is Assistant Professor of Social Work at Trinity College Dublin, Republic of Ireland, and is also a registered social worker.

International Reflections on Approaches to Mental Health Social Work

Edited by
Malcolm Golightley and Gloria Kirwan

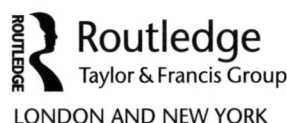

LONDON AND NEW YORK

First published 2017 by Routledge

2 Park Square, Milton Park, Abingdon, Oxfordshire OX14 4RN
711 Third Avenue, New York, NY 10017

Routledge is an imprint of the Taylor & Francis Group, an informa business

First issued in paperback 2018

British Library Cataloguing in Publication Data
A catalogue record for this book is available from the British Library

ISBN 13: 978-1-138-20299-3 (hbk)
ISBN 13: 978-0-367-02953-1 (pbk)

Typeset in Perpetua
by RefineCatch Limited, Bungay, Suffolk

Publisher's Note
The publisher accepts responsibility for any inconsistencies that may have
arisen during the conversion of this book from journal articles to book chapters,
namely the possible inclusion of journal terminology.

Disclaimer
Every effort has been made to contact copyright holders for their permission to
reprint material in this book. The publishers would be grateful to hear from any
copyright holder who is not here acknowledged and will undertake to rectify
any errors or omissions in future editions of this book.

Contents

Citation Information   vii

Notes on Contributors   ix

Introduction: mental health an issue for everyone?   1
Malcolm Golightley and Gloria Kirwan

1. Social workers' narratives of integrating mindfulness into practice   7
Robyn Lynn and Jo Mensinga

2. Early onset schizophrenia and school social work   23
Ya-Ling Chen, Barbara Rittner, Amy Manning and Rebekah Crofford

3. Analysis of social work practice: Foucault and female body image in therapy   39
Michelle Gibson

4. Police encounters in child and youth mental health: could stigma informed crisis intervention training (CIT) for parents help?   53
Maria Liegghio and Prableen Jaswal

5. Structural and cultural factors in suicide prevention: the contrast between mainstream and Inuit approaches to understanding and preventing suicide   73
Marika Morris and Claire Crooks

6. 'Only connect' 'nearest relative's' experiences of mental health act assessments   91
Martin Stuart Smith

7. Impasses in the relationship between the psychiatric rehabilitation practitioner and the consumer: a psychodynamic perspective   107
Hanoch Yerushalmi

Index   121

Citation Information

The chapters in this book were originally published in the *Journal of Social Work Practice*, volume 29, issue 3 (September 2015). When citing this material, please use the original page numbering for each article, as follows:

Editorial

Mental health an issue for everyone?
Malcolm Golightley and Gloria Kirwan
Journal of Social Work Practice, volume 29, issue 3 (September 2015), pp. 249–253

Chapter 1

Social workers' narratives of integrating mindfulness into practice
Robyn Lynn and Jo Mensinga
Journal of Social Work Practice, volume 29, issue 3 (September 2015), pp. 255–270

Chapter 2

Early onset schizophrenia and school social work
Ya-Ling Chen, Barbara Rittner, Amy Manning and Rebekah Crofford
Journal of Social Work Practice, volume 29, issue 3 (September 2015), pp. 271–286

Chapter 3

Analysis of social work practice: Foucault and female body image in therapy
Michelle Gibson
Journal of Social Work Practice, volume 29, issue 3 (September 2015), pp. 287–299

Chapter 4

Police encounters in child and youth mental health: could stigma informed crisis intervention training (CIT) for parents help?
Maria Liegghio and Prableen Jaswal
Journal of Social Work Practice, volume 29, issue 3 (September 2015), pp. 301–319

Chapter 5

Structural and cultural factors in suicide prevention: the contrast between mainstream and Inuit approaches to understanding and preventing suicide
Marika Morris and Claire Crooks
Journal of Social Work Practice, volume 29, issue 3 (September 2015), pp. 321–338

Chapter 6

'Only connect' 'nearest relative's' experiences of mental health act assessments
Martin Stuart Smith
Journal of Social Work Practice, volume 29, issue 3 (September 2015), pp. 339–353

Chapter 7

Impasses in the relationship between the psychiatric rehabilitation practitioner and the consumer: a psychodynamic perspective
Hanoch Yerushalmi
Journal of Social Work Practice, volume 29, issue 3 (September 2015), pp. 355–368

For any permission-related enquiries please visit:
http://www.tandfonline.com/page/help/permissions

Notes on Contributors

Ya-Ling Chen is a Researcher in the Department of Social Work, Chaoyang University of Technology, Taichung, Taiwan.

Rebekah Crofford, PhD, is Professor of Social Work, Roberts Wesleyan College, Rochester, USA.

Claire Crooks, PhD, is Director of School Mental Health and Associate Professor. Her research focuses on evidence-based violence prevention and mental health promotion with youth, with a particular interest in strength-based approaches with Indigenous youth and communities.

Michelle Gibson is a PhD candidate in the School of Social Work at McMaster University. Her research speciality is women's body image experience and for her dissertation she explores the intersection of HIV and embodied experience.

Malcolm Golightley is Professor of Social Work at the University of Lincoln, UK, and a registered social worker with extensive mental health experience. He is the editor of the *British Journal of Social Work*.

Prableen Jaswal is an M.S.W. student in the School of Social Work, York University, Toronto, Canada.

Gloria Kirwan is Assistant Professor of Social Work at Trinity College Dublin, Republic of Ireland, and is also a registered social worker.

Maria Liegghio is Assistant Professor in the School of Social Work, York University, Toronto, Canada.

Robyn Lynn is a Lecturer in Social Work at James Cook University, Cairns, Australia.

Amy Manning is Project Manager at the Buffalo Centre for Social Research, Buffalo, USA.

Jo Mensinga is a Lecturer in Social Work at James Cook University, Cairns, Australia.

Marika Morris, PhD, is a Canadian Institutes of Health Research Postdoctoral Fellow and an experienced community-based researcher with expertise in research with vulnerable populations and engaging in research with Indigenous, social housing and women's organizations.

Barbara Rittner is Associate Professor and Associate Dean for Advancement in the Department of Social Work, University at Buffalo, Buffalo, USA.

Martin Stuart Smith currently works as an AMHP and has worked as a social worker in the mental health field since 1984. He is particularly interested in the role of the nearest relative in relation to the Mental Health Act 1983.

Hanoch Yerushalmi, PhD, is an Associate Professor and Chair at the Department of Community Mental Health of the University of Haifa, Israel. He has been the Director of the Student Counseling Center at Hebrew University, Israel, and published articles in the areas of supervision of relational psychodynamic therapy, rehabilitation and psychoanalysis and training of clinicians.

INTRODUCTION

MENTAL HEALTH AN ISSUE FOR EVERYONE?

Mental health is a topic well worthy of a special issue of this Journal. As the dust settles over the number of articles submitted and we have had to make the choice of accepting some and not others, it by happenstance has coincided with the general election in the UK. The choice of who to govern the country and which policies have found popular favour would on the face of it provide editors with rich policy pickings. But if that was your thoughts then you would be wrong as sadly mental health services was not the prime issue and indeed mental health although mentioned never seemed to have the gravitas it deserved.

Now that the country has settled on a majority Tory government somewhat right of centre a quick read of the key public sector policies is hardly more illuminating. Mental health waiting times are to be subject to targets and this will be applied across the sector. However, apart from this, there is little or no mention of what actually happens in the interaction between the person with mental health issues and the professional from whom they are seeking help. You may find this strange as it is fairly well accepted that mental health or lack of it will affect a sizeable number of people from all walks of life and perhaps up to one in four of us will experience mental health problems at some point in our lives.

The lack of positive policies towards mental health services and the impact of cuts in public sector funding have created an abyss of indifference. Yet, as social workers we are privy to the backstage life of many who present with mental health problems and to learn what is important to them is by and large the same things that are important to us all. One of these is the centrality of relationships, with anybody but certainly with somebody. This may be therapeutic or it may simply be supportive and on occasion some relationships can be destructive. One of the characteristics of some people with mental health issues is the absence of a confiding relationship. Social workers can provide positive healing relationships and sometimes be the person (in the UK) who recommends admission to psychiatric hospital when deemed necessary.

"All human beings are born free and equal in dignity and rights" (United Nations, 1948). So reads the first line of Article 1 of the Universal Declaration of Human Rights (UDCR). As we know too well, however, across the lifespan there are many instances where individual freedoms and rights may be curtailed and compromised in many different ways. Social work increasingly seeks to position itself as working on behalf of those who find themselves disempowered, alienated or rejected by mainstream society. It is no coincidence that, in the IFSW Global Agenda for Social Work and Social Development, one of the four key priority areas for social work rallies social workers to work to uphold the "dignity and worth of the person" (Jones & Truell, 2012), thus echoing the guiding sentiment expressed in that first clause of the UDCR.

Social workers based in mental health services are faced each day with the complexities of trying to carry out such aspirational objectives, through their work to empower and support service users who as a group experience marginalization, stigma and prejudice within the wider social context. Many mental health service users will also have experienced the deprivation of their liberty under mental health legislation at one or more points in time due to concerns about their safety or that of others. The mental health social work role is mediated, therefore, within a highly charged and tension-laden social context and one in which the dominancy of the risk agenda overshadows any commitment to freedom and equality. While care in the community is a current policy and service driver, the power imbalances between providers and users of mental health services continue to intercept and arguably curtail the emancipatory and empowerment focus of social work practice in this field.

It is essential that social workers involved in this area of practice stay attuned to the competing discourses and values that surround and influence their work. The impetus for this special edition of the Journal was grounded in the view that social workers benefit from knowing about the experience of social workers in different local contexts against which they can compare and contrast their own experiences and practice.

We are delighted that the call for articles drew responses from social workers engaged in mental health practice across the world. We are aware that there is no homogenous social work response in this field and that context and culture play their parts in shaping the role of social workers in responding to the needs of mental health service users and informal carers in different localities. However, we believe that sharing information, perspectives, dilemmas and concerns across boundaries and borders serves to inform and enhance local social work practice. In a rapidly changing context, both local and international, social workers are working to respond to need very often in risk-focused and risk-averse contexts, where promoting individual freedom and dignity competes with the interests of the 'greater good' or is constrained due to lack of resource investment. In working to make social institutions, local and international, more responsive to the needs of people with mental health difficulties, social workers will encounter tensions between theoretical aspirations and the realities of practice. They need as many outlets as possible to exchange and learn from each other's experiences. In *Squarings*, Seamus Heaney writes, "the places I go back to have not failed but will not last" (Heaney, 2014, p. 53) and likewise mental health social work must find ways to share "what works" while at the same time looking to the future development of this field of practice. We hope this special edition can modestly contribute to such an exchange and possibly prompt some further discussions on how to maintain a vibrancy and sense of renewal in mental health social work practice.

The annual UK mental health awareness week has also passed by and mindfulness was the topic chosen for this year's focus. Several promotions were held throughout the country and concerted efforts seemed to have been made to promote mental health awareness throughout the general population. There is a danger that 'mindfulness' becomes little more than the latest current fashion practised by social workers who have a brief understanding and training in this approach. We thought it especially relevant to incorporate an original article that draws on some research to explore mindfulness. Sitting alongside other original articles, this special issue illustrates the breadth of work in mental health and interesting issues from different cultural contexts.

Robyn Lynn and Jo Mensinga in their article "Social workers' narratives of integrating mindfulness into practice" draw our attention to Eastern origins of the practice of mindfulness. Their article owes much to the critiques that student social workers and practitioners made of the practice of mindfulness and as they saw it the tension between value-based practice and therapy. The process of incorporating mindfulness into practice meant reconciling the participant's personal and professional discourse within their developing knowledge base. In part, this was due to the nature of transporting a practice rooted in eastern practice to a western approach that required the practitioner to merge these different world views with their individual approach to social work. This article really does add to the debate and provides a useful foil to the uncritical acceptance of what could be dismissed by some as the latest fad in therapy.

Ya Ling Chen, Barbara Rittner, Amy Manning and Rebekah Crofford provide us with a thought-provoking article on the controversial subject of the diagnosis and the subsequent response of children and young people with schizophrenia. The idea that children could be diagnosed as having schizophrenia provokes argument and discussion, and while this is rare it raises fascinating and interesting glimpses into just what it is that we call these behaviours in children and young people. Writing from the USA cultural context, the article reviews prevalence rates and the controversy over diagnosis in children and adolescents. That this is manifest in poor achievement at school should come as no surprise although interesting to read and a reminder of the important role that social workers based in schools can have. The USA context also raises serious issues about the financial, social and emotional stress that a diagnosis of a major psychosis can produce. Adjustments in the home and school are central to this but, in addition, there is the issue of health insurance coverage, which may be dependent upon a psychiatric diagnosis.

It would have been hard to produce a special issue without at least a passing mention to Foucault and we are fortunate that Michelle Gibson has produced an interesting article on social work practice and Foucault and the female body image. She presents a powerful argument for looking beyond the limitations of the CBT approach with its emphasis on the individual to incorporate socio-political perspectives. Writing from a personal and professional viewpoint, Gibson explores her own reactions to the pressure placed on women by a society with a narrow and often one-dimensional view about beauty and health and body image. Social workers are caught up in this and through uncritical approaches may be reinforcing unhealthy messages. Gibson produces an analysis of the present psychological model of treatment of body image dissatisfaction from a Foucauldian perspective and in so doing offers an alternative of critical practice that facilitates both the client and worker to develop a more honest therapeutic relationship.

Maria Liegghio and Prableen Jaswal explore the dynamics surrounding the involvement of police personnel in mental health crisis situations, where police assistance is sought by a family member or carer to help deal with the distressed behaviour of a young person. This article, based on the findings emerging from a Canadian research study, illuminates the frequency and intensity of situations in which police personnel are called in to de-escalate situations related to a young person's mental distress. Oftentimes, these situations involve highly charged and conflictual scenarios taking place in a family context and where parents or carers feel unable to manage the young person's behaviour without external assistance. The implications for young people with mental health problems of this type of contact with law enforcement services is explored and the article promotes the benefits of crisis intervention training for family members with the aim of reducing the need for this type of police intervention.

The article by Marika Morris and Claire Crooks not only deals with the very serious topic of suicide in contemporary society, but it also highlights in considerable detail the history of the Inuit people and their struggle to survive decades of destructive and oppressive social policies, including family separation and the loss of cultural identity and traditions. This article provides a careful analysis of documentary evidence, which demonstrates how the rise in suicide among the Inuit must be understood within the context of racist, and oppressive policies, which this population has endured over recent generations. The picture that emerges of disrupted families, alienated communities and the loss of cultural identity highlights the influence that structural factors can have on suicide rates within a population. While awareness of individual risk factors is always relevant, this very detailed article emphasizes the societal influences, which can be significant but often invisible in their impact on suicidal ideation and rates of completed suicides. For social work practitioners, this article serves as a serious reminder of the need to pay attention to the wider social context of individual distress.

Mental health social work in the UK is never far from issues around compulsory admission to hospital and in the article "Only Connect" Martin Smith looks at the importance of the nearest relative, a specific term defined in the Mental Health legislation. Examining in depth the experiences of the nearest relative in relation to the compulsory admission decision, it becomes clear that the relationship between the social worker (Approved Mental Health Professional) and the nearest relative and the service user is a significant predictor of the levels of satisfaction that the nearest relative reports. This should come as no surprise as one of the impacts of mental illness is a feeling of isolation and a lack of understanding about the nature of the mental illness and the processes that become involved. The qualities of empathy, explanation, understanding, caring and support are especially valued in the process and social workers need to use their relationship building skills to create situations where these qualities are enhanced.

Hanoch Yerushalmi in his article, based in Israel, takes a psychodynamic perspective when examining breakdowns in service user and practitioner relationships and the impact that this can have on rehabilitation from serious mental illness. This relationship he writes is crucial for recovery and may be used by the service user as a role model on which to develop other significant relationships. He makes the case that the rupture in the relationship can occur when the practitioner is not fully alert to the service user's needs and that the impasse in the relationship may also reflect previous experiences of the service user. Using insights from the therapeutic field, it is possible that he suggests to adapt and respond to impasses in the professional relationship. He provides some illustrative and helpful examples of when an impasse in the professional relationship has occurred and how through empathetic and emotional investment the professional relationship can be strengthened and even developed.

As usual for this Journal, we have included two reviews of books and selected ones that we think are especially relevant to this special issue and compliment each other. Juliet Koprowska discusses William R. Miller and Stephen Rollnick's (2013) book, *Motivational Interviewing* which is now in its third edition and takes into account the numerous research studies into motivational interviewing, some more positive than others but all approached in this text with a degree of honesty and helpful assessment. Koprowska concludes that this book provides a valuable contribution to a developing understand of MI as a helping process.

Our final book review is by Claire Gregor and she read Melinda Hohman (2012), *Motivational interviewing in social work practice,* which is intended to complement the book reviewed by Juliet Koprowska in this issue. Written from a largely USA perspective, the book includes extracts from service user interviews and the rider that motivational interviewing skills are not simple to learn and may require additional ongoing training and support. Gregor concludes that this is a very accessible text that in her opinion would be more of an additional text rather than core reading.

References

Heaney, S. (2014) *'Squarings: xli', Seamus Heaney: new selected poems 1988–2013*, Faber & Faber, London.

Hohman, M. (2012) *Motivational Interviewing in Social Work Practice*, Guilford Press, New York.

Jones, D. & Truell, R. (2012) 'The global agenda for social work and social development: a place to link together and be effective in a globalized world', *International Social Work*, vol. 55, no. 4, pp. 454–472.

Miller, W. R. & Rollnick, S. (2013) *Motivational Interviewing* (3rd ed), Guilford Press, New York.

United Nations (1948) *Universal declaration of human rights*. Available at: http://www.un.org/en/documents/udhr/index.shtml

Malcolm Golightley
University of Lincoln, School of health and Social Care,
Bridge House, Brayford, Lincoln, United Kingdom

Gloria Kirwan
Trinity College Dublin, Dublin, Ireland

Robyn Lynn and Jo Mensinga

SOCIAL WORKERS' NARRATIVES OF INTEGRATING MINDFULNESS INTO PRACTICE

Mindfulness is increasingly important as a professional intervention in social work; however, little is known about how practitioners integrate a practice of eastern origins into a western context. To explore the integration of mindfulness in social work, we collected written stories from social workers who participated in two workshops in regional Australia. The participants developed their own individual written narratives about their understanding of and experience in using mindfulness, and contributed these to a larger group discussion. We identified four scenarios/plotlines within the collected stories and 'restoried' four examples of the participants' written narratives. The stories reveal that participants experience little dissonance when integrating mindfulness into their personal lives, but the process of incorporating it into their practice requires a complex negotiation between the participant's story of themselves as a practitioner of mindfulness, their 'professional story', stories of themselves as social workers and the story of social work in their professional knowledge landscape.

Introduction

Mindfulness is increasingly being researched and adopted in psychology, medicine and education, and has recently become more prominent in the social work literature. It is commonly defined as 'moment-to-moment awareness' or 'paying attention to the moment without judgement' and encourages attention to every movement, breath, feeling and thought – a 'consciousness alive to the present reality' (Hanh, 1976, p. 11).

In social work, the primary means of cultivating mindfulness is through formal and informal meditation practices and mindfulness-based applications. Although often associated with spiritual traditions, mindfulness can be learnt in a secular context without the support of a religion, as a means of facilitating awareness of the present moment (Hick, 2009, p. 2). This present moment orientation has been shown to be of benefit at the individual, group and community levels in social work, particularly in the development of increased attention, heightened self- awareness, cultivation of empathy and compassion, inner calm and peace, more insight and transformative ways of living and being (Coholic, 2005; Berceli & Napoli, 2006; Minor & Carlson, 2006; Hick, 2009).

As academics, we have included aspects of mindfulness and embodied awareness into our teaching in the university sector (Mensinga, 2010, 2011). However, following student questions and challenges about the value base underpinning these techniques, we developed an interest in exploring what, if any, ethical issues and/or dilemmas could arise when introducing mindfulness into social work practice settings. In another paper, we investigated the question 'is mindfulness value free?' and the implications (if any) for practitioners in the sector (Lynn, Mensinga, Tinning, & Lundman, 2015). During this inquiry, we found that issues and tensions that arose were largely due to a perceived conflict of interest between the orientation and approach to practice, advocated by the social work profession and the workers' own experiences, training and understanding of mindfulness (Lynn *et al.*, 2015). We concluded that while mindfulness has been shown to be a natural process that can be cultivated, its translation and evolution as an eastern practice into a western context requires the worker to merge different cultural and world views while also integrating their own personal experience into what they perceive as the espoused orientation and approach of the social work profession.

Healy contends that social workers' 'knowledge, purpose and skills bases - are substantially constructed in, and through, the environments in which [they] work' (2005, p. 4). Although this professional knowledge context is a 'dominant story' that is itself a part and parcel of the larger discourse that determines 'what is a profession', we began to wonder if the eastern origins of mindfulness actually mattered to social workers' as they came to know about and chose to use mindfulness in practice. Drawing on Fenstermacher's work (1994), whose interest was in the epistemological drivers underpinning knowledge creation in education, we identified four questions, we thought would help us address our concerns and help us better understand the process by which social workers integrated mindfulness into their practice:

- How do social workers come to know about mindfulness?
- What do social workers know about the effective use of mindfulness in social work?
- What knowledge do social workers consider essential for using mindfulness?
- Who do social workers trust to produce knowledge about mindfulness in social work?

With these questions in mind, we designed and delivered two workshops in two different regional cities along the East coast of Australia. The workshops provided a space for two separate groups of social workers to develop their own individual written narratives about mindfulness and to reflect on them in a larger group discussion. Following the workshop, we engaged in a process of focused reading of the written stories and reviewed notes and transcripts of the discussions. We familiarised ourselves with all the data by initially noting our own influence on the production of the narratives before identifying existing themes. This was followed by a further analysis of the collected stories, in which we used Clandinin and Connelly's (2000) three-dimensional space approach to better understand the influences on the participating social workers' knowledge of and uptake of mindfulness in their practice.

In line with Clandinin and Connelly's (2000) narrative inquiry approach, we chose to restory and present four examples of the participants' written narratives to illustrate the dimensions/influence of place, time and social interaction made explicit during the workshops. In doing so, we revealed that the contextual nature of the profession as described by Healy (2005) and what we named the 'professional story' does indeed impact the process by which social workers story the acquisition of and use of mindfulness in practice. Similarly, in the process of exploring the four questions we raised in relationship with Fenstermacher's (1994) epistemological drivers, we conclude that the integration of mindfulness into social work practice is both a contextual and relational process that draws on the practitioner's personal experience/knowledge of mindfulness (rather than on its religious underpinnings or theoretical understandings) and is influenced by their assessment of clients' needs within the agency context.

Mindfulness in social work

Interest in mindfulness in social work is a relatively recent phenomenon that is not fully integrated into the purpose, professional knowledge base and framework for practice. From the mid 2000s onwards, there have been a number of articles that indicate social work is engaging with mindfulness in individual, group and community interventions (Hick, 2009). They often use research undertaken in psychology, sociology or medicine to define and inform their knowledge of mindfulness and to provide the primary source of evidence of the effectiveness of mindfulness-based applications. These practices are used as a form of intervention, for cultivating a positive relationship with clients and as a mode of self-care for social workers and their clients (Hick & Furlotte, 2009).

Mindfulness-based applications have their roots in the Buddhist traditions that describe it as a process or spiritual practice that involves distinct phases of development (Bodhi, 2011; Milton, 2011). In western psychology, there are a range of definitions and ways of operationalising mindfulness. The emphasis in these definitions has been on what it is and how to measure and develop it (Grossman & Van Dam, 2011; Milton, 2011, p. 24). These more recent accounts that have evolved through the science of mindfulness differ considerably from the traditional way it was defined. The recognition of these differences has led to an increase in discussion about whether the separation of mindfulness from its holistic roots in this work is useful and/or appropriate (Grossman & Van Dam, 2011; Wallace, 2006, 2011).

Hick and Furlotte (2009) in their review of the definitions of mindfulness in social work identify Bishop et al.'s (2004) definition as the most commonly applied in social work. This definition has a health and wellness focus. Bishop et al. describe mindfulness as a two component model consisting of (a) 'self-regulation of attention so that it is maintained on immediate experience, thereby allowing for increased recognition of mental events in the present moment', and (b) 'adopting a particular orientation toward one's experiences in the present moment...characterized by curiosity, openness, and acceptance' (2004, p. 232). Drawing on this or similar definitions and knowledge from other sciences, the social work literature is beginning to develop its own theoretical, factual and practical knowledge (Trevithick, 2008) about the role and effectiveness of mindfulness for the social worker and the people with whom they work (Birnbaum & Birnbaum, 2008; Hick, 2008, 2009; Hick & Furlotte, 2009; Lee *et al.*, 2009, Turner, 2009; Gause and Coholic, 2010; Segal *et al.*, 2010) While it is important to generate this knowledge in the context of social work, we propose that this is only part of the story about social workers' knowledge and use of mindfulness and that an exploration of how they come to know about and integrate mindfulness practices is also necessary.

The 'professional story' of social work

Like other professions, social work lays claim to a particular way of knowing reality that forms part of a 'sacred story' on a professional knowledge landscape (Clandinin & Connolly, 1996). In the case of social work, this story attempts to gloss over its religious-linked beginnings and adopt a materialist-positivist world view that both fosters a preferred humanist-modernist professional paradigm and helps to lay claim to knowledge and skills considered unique to social work (Payne, 1996; Fook *et al.*, 2000; Fook, 2002; Lynn, 2010). However, what constitutes social work knowledge still remains inconclusive. While some authors choose to emphasise scientific, rational and legitimate knowledge, others focus on action and experience (Trevithick, 2008). Healy (2005), on the other hand, draws attention to a *constructed knowledge space* where the knowledge social workers assume to inform their *purpose and practice* is constantly negotiated between the different components that make up this space.

For our purposes then, we adopted Healy's (2005) model as a preferred way of understanding social work knowledge. We believed that Healy's (2005) concept of a constructed knowledge space better captured the challenges that practitioners would encounter when trying to integrate mindfulness into practice. The model itself identifies the practitioner's need to consider the *institutional context* (including public policies, laws, organisational policies as well as accepted practices); the *formal professional base* (service discourses from the human sciences, formal theories of practice, Judeo-Christian beliefs and formally accepted skills) and the worker's own *individual framework* (practice wisdom, developed theories of professional practice and skills and acquired knowledge) when actioning a particular practice approach. In our reckoning, then when choosing to adopt mindfulness, the social worker would not only need to reconcile their own experience of mindfulness within a western cultural context, but they would also need to navigate the dominant discourses that are strongly related to the materialist/positivist, humanist and modernist principles of objectivity, rationality and individualism which influence what is considered to be the appropriate knowledge for practice and practice decisions (Healy, 2005; Bell, 2012).

Clandinin and Connelly (1995) describe a similar process as that outlined by Healy (2005) when exploring how teachers made sense of presenting demands to negotiate their *purpose and practice* of teaching. However, in their work they propose that this process is best understood narratively and by way of metaphor. They suggest the image of a 'professional knowledge landscape' to depict the space in which teachers tell stories to account for their professional practice and understand the stories told in that space as the means by which teachers traverse the landscape. Drawing on both Clandinin and Connelly (1995) and Healy's (2005) work as ways to understand the integration of mindfulness into social workers' practice, we decided that collecting and exploring the stories social workers told about how they came to learn about and implemented mindfulness in their practice would provide answers to our questions as outlined in the beginning of this paper.

Preparing for and hosting 'A conversation about mindfulness in social work'

Our project was conducted at a regional university in Australia as part of its field education professional development program. The project was designed with the dual purpose of providing a professional development opportunity for social workers interested in participating in 'A conversation about mindfulness in social work', while at the same time producing material for our research on the inclusion of mindfulness approaches into social work practice.

The Social Work Field Education Unit invited social workers on their database to two professional development workshops. Each workshop was aimed at social workers who were familiar with mindfulness and who had either adopted it or were interested in its application in practice. On receiving Ethics Approval, interested participants were sent an information sheet which invited them to take part in our research on mindfulness in social work as part of their attendance. This information also outlined the aims of the research, data collection and management processes, the voluntary nature of participation, confidentiality and how the findings would be disseminated.

The workshops, of three hours duration, were held in two regional centres in Australia. The stated aims for the workshops were (a) to facilitate and collect participants' individual written narratives about their use (or desired use) of mindfulness in social work; (b) to provide a safe space in which participants could critically reflect upon and discuss their narrative and its meaning for their practice; (c) to develop a shared understanding of the possible tensions and dilemmas that may arise when using mindfulness, particularly in light of the ethics and values espoused by the profession, and (d) to identify any emerging implications for practice.

Each workshop began with some yoga and meditation practice. Information about the research aspect of the workshop was then revisited and formal consent sought to record and use participants' written narratives and conversations from the workshop. All of the participants provided consent. Nine participants engaged in one workshop and eight in the other. Seven participants in each of the workshops had adopted mindfulness into their work and wanted to further develop their use of it in their practice. Only three of the total participants had not had the opportunity to use meditation. Participants were from a range of government and non-government organisations.

At the beginning of each workshop, we identified ourselves as 'curious participants' rather than 'knowledge holders'. Although we hoped to elicit and engage with all the 'knowledge and experience' related to mindfulness in the room, being academics, we were aware of the possibility of inhibiting the conversation. Jo is a practitioner and teacher of yoga who at the time was the Field Education Coordinator and so knew some of the participants in the context of field placement organisation and support. Robyn practices Buddhist meditation. Though she had no specific role in field education, Robyn knew some of the participants in one of the workshops as fellow social workers. We were also aware that the stories were being written and collected as a professional development activity and this could potentially impact how the participants responded to the task of writing their practice stories.

Once introductions were completed, participants were given 15 minutes to write a story about their experience of mindfulness in practice. No definition of mindfulness was provided by us as we were interested in the participants' own understandings and believed these would emerge in the stories they told about the way they integrated mindfulness into their practice. However the 'Tree of Contemplative Practice' (see Figure 1) from the Centre for Contemplative Mind in Society was introduced to the participants before writing their stories to stimulate their thinking about and reflection on their own lived story of mindfulness practices. The tree provided participants with a

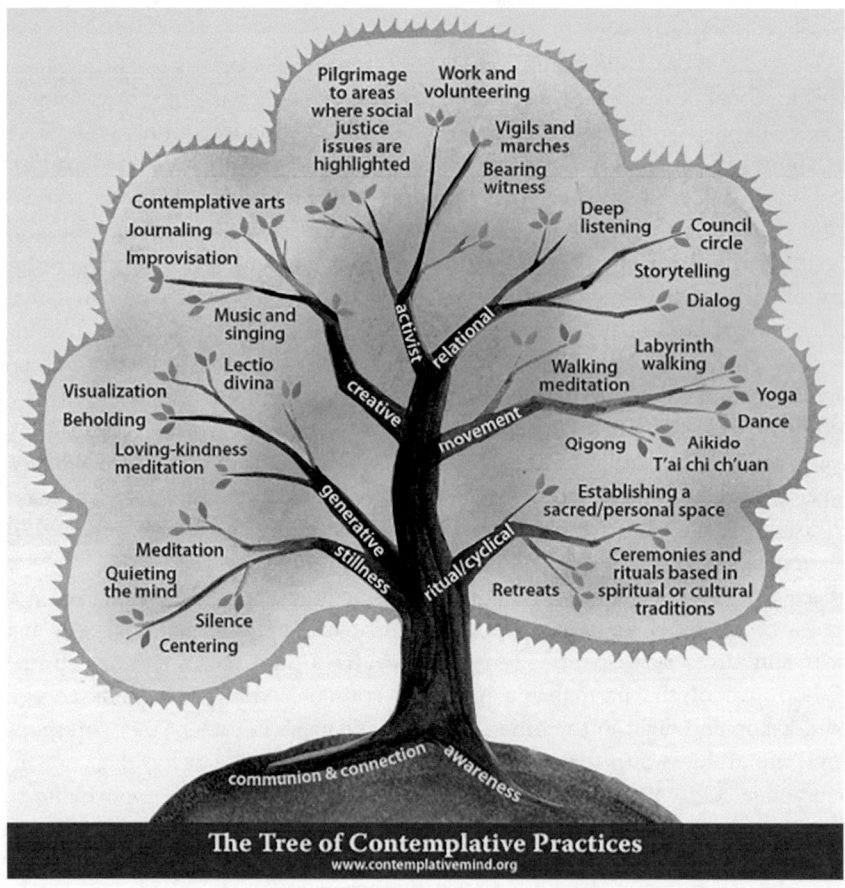

FIGURE 1 Tree of Contemplative Practices (http://www.contemplativemind.org/practices/tree.html)

visual image of various contemplative practices. The roots of the tree symbolise the intention of the practices (communion, connection and awareness), while the branches represent different approaches that can be adopted to facilitate contemplation such as stillness, creativity or movement. This contributed to a broader understanding of mindfulness that could have had an effect on their individual definitions of mindfulness. We also provided four questions to stimulate their thinking: (1) what is your understanding of mindfulness? (2) how did you arrive at that understanding? (3) how did you use it in your practice? and (4) what tensions or ethical dilemmas do you encounter in integrating it into your practice?

Exploring the collected stories of mindfulness

Following the workshops, on two separate occasions, we each individually read all of the written narratives and then came together to share our understandings. On the first reading, we focused on the nature of the stories, exploring how our own position as workshop facilitators and as practitioner academics may have impacted the narratives (Riessmann, 2007). We also sought to identify any possible influence that the context and the workshop agenda may have had on the type of stories the practitioners wrote. During the second reading, we individually identified common themes and then came together to combine and mind map our responses. This led to a third analysis phase where we returned to Clandinin and Connelly's (1995) metaphor of a professional knowledge landscape and drew on Ollerenshaw and Creswell's (2002) summary of the key aspects of Clandinin and Connelly's (2000) three-dimensional space approach to analyse the practitioner narratives in more detail.

On our first reading, we were both struck by how the questions we had provided had influenced the way the participants had written their stories, and concluded that we too had been influenced by the 'professional story' when constructing the workshop. For example, the questions we provided for stimulation reflected the significance of the contextual nature of social work. We also noticed that when the participants wrote their stories, many tended to address the questions rather than use them as a source of stimulation for their thinking about their own larger story. In fact, rather than provide a 'whole' story, the written narratives consisted of fragmented descriptions of events, happenings and experiences – much like case notes or responses to short answer questions in an exam. Nevertheless, what at first seemed to be disjointed pieces of writing with no beginning, middle or end, on a closer reading emerged as 'big and small stories' (Bamberg, 2006) of mindfulness in social work. The effect of the Tree of Contemplative Practice, if any, on the quality of their stories was not clear. Following our second reading, we identified four main scenarios or plotlines emerging from the stories: mindfulness as a practice; mindfulness as a social construct; mindfulness as a negotiated practice and ethical issues associated with introducing mindfulness.

To better understand how these 'plotlines' assisted the participants to integrate mindfulness into their practice, we again revisited the stories and noticed that the linking of knowledge, context and identity within a particular space, place and time was important in both the practitioner's personal and/or professional experience. The emerging relationship between space, place and time prompted a final analysis where

(Robyn) followed Ollerenshaw and Creswell's (2002) summary of Clandinin and Connelly's (2000) three-dimensional space approach to analyse the practitioner narratives. This approach enabled us to focus on the broader wholistic experience of the participants that was central in their stories and involved analysing the following elements in the individual participant stories: (i) personal and social interaction with others; (ii) continuity of past, present and future experiences and (iii) any specific situations or places in their experience (Clandinin & Connelly, 2000). The initial three-dimensional space narrative structure was then shared with (Jo) who reviewed the analysis. Through this process, we formed a new story that highlights the experiences and interactions that occurred in their narratives of mindfulness.

However, a limitation of this approach is that it continues in the tradition of using western empirical scientific methods to explore the use of mindfulness in social work. These methods retain the mind/body split that exist within the modernist 'professional story' of social work (Mensinga, 2011) and hinder any significant ontological and epistemological shift occurring in social work. It is only with more emphasis given to the empiricism of the visceral (Mensinga, 2011) and the contemplative or consciousness disciplines (Wallace, 2012) that the subjectively experienced mental states and processes that occur in the use of mindfulness in social work can become part of research observations and contribute to a real paradigm shift in social work.

Narrative plotlines emerging from the stories of mindfulness in social work

Consistent with Clandinin and Connelly's (2000) approach, we present our findings as a number of stories to illustrate the scenarios/plotlines we identified as the means that social workers use to navigate within the 'professional story' on the professional landscape. Moreover, like all the stories told and written in the workshop, these examples also provide insights into how social workers' knowledge of mindfulness involves the linking of knowledge, context and identity within a particular space, place and time in the practitioner's personal and professional life. While the stories presented here are based on fact, they are also 'fictionalised'. That is, the names and order of events within each of the identified plotlines have been reconstructed from the fragmented stories we collected. This process provides narrative coherence while maintaining confidentiality for the participants.

Mindfulness is both a practice and a social construct

Mari's story

> I came to understand mindfulness through my own personal experience of trauma and awareness. I began by walking. I remember the pleasure of walking around on soft grass with no shoes for ten minutes a day and how it was an escape from the pain and struggle of postnatal depression. It helped me to stop listening to my depressed thoughts and voices and instead I began to listen to my breath, my body, to feel the sun on my skin and become more aware of colours, touch, and smells.

I don't use walking as a practice anymore. Instead I enjoy visualisations and experience mindfulness as a way of being 'conscious'. But it was because of my initial experience and how it helped me that I still use mindfulness today and have shared various practices with my own children and with clients in the workplace.

Professionally I draw on my personal experience when working with traumatised clients - especially with those who have underlying anxiety and PTSD. However, with them, I prefer to use art as a tool rather than other practices as I don't think the clients would feel safe if I asked them to close their eyes. When using art I aim to develop awareness and often give feedback on what I see and hear in my interactions with the client. For example, I might draw their attention to a grimace they have just made. Hmmm, as an aside though, I have noticed that clients who are what I call 'indoctrinated Christians' are wary of mindfulness.

Morgans's story

I became interested in mindfulness practices during the 1970s. I used to join a group of actors and dancers who would do yoga for the first hour of their daily class at University. Yoga became part of my personal life – I even took up fasting on a weekly basis for 3 years. However, it was when I lived in India and Papua New Guinea and became immersed in many of their cultural practices that I found that my own practice deepened. In India I would join the host where I lived when she did yoga and meditation – something she did for three hours each day. During this time I learnt to focus more on breathing and how to build a relationship with it and then integrate it with how I ate. I also used my focus on the breath as a way of living and relating to others. In Papua New Guinea the chanting and singing that women engaged in to ward off spirits and strengthen the community provided another experience of mindfulness for me. For me then, mindfulness has become a practice of focused awareness that is nurturing and is experienced through centring and inner stillness, reflection, and meditation (which can include breathing/yoga).

In my experience mindfulness is a cultural practice that can be adapted within our own. Although I am very aware of the 'new age' links that some people/ clients can attach to mindfulness and that the practices themselves originate from Hindu/Buddhist religions, I believe that the techniques can be utilized within the professional context of social work. I liken it to the fact that personally and as a culture I am [we are] quite happy to eat pasta, which is an Italian food from a mainly Catholic country, and curry from India. And I don't see this as being any different. In my professional practice then, if in my assessment I think the client and situation could benefit from the introduction of centring, reflection and/or meditation I will incorporate breathing, meditation, visualization and/or deep listening into my therapy with them. It's interesting though, even though at one level I don't have any real ethical dilemmas about the use of mindfulness in social work, at another level I do think that I need to engage in more exploration of the ethical dilemmas that could arise.

These stories illustrate how these two practitioners have drawn on their own personal experience to inform their professional practice. The importance of experience as a source of knowledge is not an untold story within either the 'knowledge base' of social work (Drury Hudson, 1997; Trevithick, 2008) nor within that connected with the use of mindfulness in social work (Hick, 2008). Both Mari and Morgan came to see mindfulness as a personal/natural way of being that is useful to the well-being of themselves and their clients and consider it a personal or cultural practice that can be integrated into one's professional life or cultural practices. They saw mindfulness both as a practice and a social construct. This is reflected in the connections they made between how they were introduced to mindfulness and how they justified its use in their practice. Mari's own experience of understanding trauma and developing awareness through her body (Mensinga, 2011) informed her use of mindfulness in trauma/awareness work in her practice. Morgan's experience of it as a cultural practice was adapted and incorporated into the cultural context of social work. In both stories, the use of mindfulness in the professional context is monitored according to client characteristics and the participants' practice wisdom within the context of the 'professional story' (Healy, 2005).

Mindfulness as a negotiated practice

Lucy's story

> I learnt about mindfulness through my own exploration of contemplative practices and the positive and negative challenges I have faced in life. My earliest experience would have been as a child, at Sunday School where I learnt about prayer and 'nonprayer'. Later I explored yoga, meditation, journaling, and different forms of spirituality and even immersed myself in a vegan lifestyle. I also remember learning 'if this happens, then . . . breathe, listen, feel'. Through these experiences I came to understand mindfulness as 'being there in the moment' - letting myself listen without cross examining my intuitive/gut feelings; acknowledging and accepting rather than trying to diagnose or jump forward before the moment has been fully experienced or lived. In doing so, I consciously enjoy the moment and am aware of the feelings and experience - being still and calm in the busyness or chaos of life. It is part of who I am. It helps me to survive.
>
> I take this understanding into the workplace and have engaged in a number of different activities with clients. For instance I have included drawing to various types of music; creative journaling with clients in a sexual assault service; a mindfulness exercise using Easter eggs with students; teaching clients to count backwards from 21 (in 3s); going to a happy place with deep breathing; and giving my full attention and focus so the other person knows that they are heard. I also think my practice has helped me in my ability to empathise and have respect – person to person rather than client to worker/'expert' – cultivating equality rather than reinforcing a power imbalance. In fact, I think it is through listening (more), talking (less), listening (more than before), talking (less than before) and giving space for the words, I have learnt never to underestimate the capacity of others to find their solution.

However, although I think of mindfulness as a 'halo' around my professional practice I do ask myself 'do I really know what I'm doing?' While I always consider things like the client's age, cognitive ability, and their willingness to participate in these activities- particularly as I currently work with involuntary clients who are mandated and/or court ordered – there are a number of questions that I also find myself asking. What is the stance of the professional accrediting body? Does this fit with the framework of the service? If it doesn't, is this able to change and if not am I then practising in an unethical manner? I think it is also made more difficult when my framework is not fully understood or valued by colleagues or supervisors in the sector. But there are also other difficulties- time and trying to slow things down in the current service/system is so hard. I am so aware of the competing requirements of completing 'tasks' and wanting to engage in an experience with my clients.

Lucy's story, like Mari's and Morgan's, still lies with the personal. However, while Lucy described meditation as a 'halo' around her practice, unlike the others she struggles with the implementation of it in her professional knowledge landscape. Mindfulness in her context is a negotiated practice that is more of a 'secret story' (Clandinin & Connelly, 1996) about her work - not fully known, understood or valued by her colleagues and supervisors. Her story raises the importance of the 'professional story' and her struggle to reconcile professional knowledge, context and identity.

The ethical practice of mindfulness

David's story

Mindfulness allows me to be present in the moment, taking each moment as it comes. I describe it as a feeling of being merged with 'Brahman' (the source of power and eternity), which brings me peace within. However being able to achieve this state is difficult. Still, I believe it has great potential for us in our contemporary lives because people by nature would like to experience calm and peace of mind in life. Mindfulness, as a process, provides this opportunity for people, especially for those who find it difficult to pay attention in the present moment.

In my own practice I use techniques that are accepted by the social work profession based on research evidence from psychology, for example, the 3 minute breathing exercise and cognitive restructuring. These exercises enable the client to experience feelings and emotions and stay with them. While useful, I do have a number of dilemmas around social workers providing services to clients without having an adequate knowledge base and/or theoretical understanding behind mindfulness interventions. Although it has its roots in Buddhism, mindfulness has been developed and incorporated into the medical field. As a consequence, I believe that many practitioners present mindfulness as a 'capsule of techniques' that doesn't capture its rich traditions and practice wisdom. After all, within the eight fold path to wisdom 'paying attention' is only one of those paths. For example, I don't see any consideration given to the question 'why is there suffering on this earth?'- a question that is central to the noble truths of Buddhism. But then this raises issues at another level. I think the social work discourse needs to rethink the bio-psycho-social-cultural model and consider whether mindfulness as an element of spirituality needs to be included. This then raises questions about the 'value of the medical model versus traditional wisdom' and 'evidence based knowledge versus religious/spiritual knowledge'. Still, I do wonder why we want to create 'evidence' when mindfulness is already known to be effective in people's lives.

David's story is one where mindfulness as a spiritual activity has been given legitimacy by its incorporation into the medical field. To justify its use, it has been melded with the dominant discourse, but David questions what is lost in its adaptation to professional and organisational discourses. He sees a need to rethink these discourses from the perspective of traditional wisdoms and religious and spiritual knowledge. His concern is with the ethical practice of mindfulness. This story is similar in some respects to Morgan and Lucy's stories of working with mindfulness within the context of the professional and organisational discourses, though it differs in that David identified aspects of the 'sacred story' of social work that need to be rethought in light of the roots of mindfulness.

How do social workers come to understand and incorporate mindfulness into practice?

In light of the stories presented, just as Healy (2005) and Clandinin and Connelly (1996) concluded in their work, it is clear that how these social workers come to know about mindfulness and integrate it into their practice cannot be understood in a few sentences. Rather, we suggest that the importance of the eastern origins of mindfulness in their practice is a complex relationship between the storyteller's story of themselves as a practitioner of mindfulness, their 'professional story', stories of themselves as social workers and the story of social work in their professional knowledge landscape. Similarly, in keeping with this assertion, the four questions we posed at the beginning need to be answered conditionally, with an 'it depends'.

In our first question we asked 'How do social workers come to know about mindfulness?' The stories, from the participants' in our conversation 'Mindfulness in Social Work', reveal a knowledge and understanding of mindfulness largely grows out of personal experience, which includes an exposure to other cultures; physical challenges and/or their own interest in developing spiritual practices within and outside of traditional religious contexts. 'How they came to know' also includes learning through the body and engaging in contemplative experiences that lie outside the materialist/positivist, humanist and modernist principles of objectivity and rationality espoused by the profession. However, the stories also reveal that this knowledge is adapted, rather than preserved, into the 'professional story' both within the context of the professional and organisational discourses that arise on particular professional knowledge landscapes. Furthermore, while stories like Morgan and David's reveal a confidence about integrating mindfulness into practice, Lucy's awareness of prevailing professional and organisational discourses mean she uses it opportunistically. We wonder whether a shift in values would encourage Lucy and others like her to no longer cosset a 'secret story' about mindfulness, but instead contribute their stories to a growing body of knowledge that can then be explored in more depth by others.

In relation to our second question *'What do social workers know about the effective use of mindfulness in social work?'* our answer of 'it depends' is even more apparent. In the stories that Mari, Morgan, Lucy and David tell about what might constitute the form and effective use of mindfulness in social work, there appears to be a direct link between the stories they tell about what it means for them to be a practitioner of mindfulness and those that reveal their understanding of the professional knowledge landscape. Similar to Healy's (2005) description of the 'professional story', their social work story of mindfulness changes within different organisations and fields. For example, the effective use of mindfulness in Lucy's story is defined more by the culture, values and norms of her organisation and those committed to valuing such work rather than by any tested knowledge base or personal practical experience. Once again, we believe that it is only by changing the dominant and service discourses and the values they foster that a practice once seen as strange or ineffectual may become valued on the professional knowledge landscape.

We suggest that the stories also indicate that a conditional 'it depends' applies to the remaining questions we have posed – i.e., w*hat knowledge do social workers consider essential for using mindfulness* and *who do social workers trust to produce knowledge about mindfulness in social work?* All four stories suggest that client characteristics' and their defined needs, the agency context and how the practitioner perceives their own social work identity determines what knowledge is essential when using mindfulness in practice. Mari, Morgan, Lucy and David also indicate a need to adapt the knowledge they had acquired from their own personal experiences when using mindfulness in their professional practice. David, for example, turned to medical sources about mindfulness as a trusted source of knowledge production to help integrate his knowledge into practice. On the other hand, David also questions this process and suggests that a deeper understanding of the epistemological underpinnings of mindfulness is just as important as modifying techniques to fit a western context. However, although there is a vast knowledge base about mindfulness in Buddhist and other religious literature and more recently an emerging knowledge base in social work that could be drawn on when introducing mindfulness in practice, the participants' stories reveal that choosing knowledge that enables them to navigate the different components of the 'professional story' is more important.

Summary and possibilities

Although the four stories presented in this article are examples of the written narratives collected in the workshops, these stories reflect the content and processes described in the remaining narratives. All the practitioners who participated in the workshops, even those who had yet to include mindfulness into their practice, noted an emerging knowledge system about mindfulness in social work and described a map of how social workers move through and responsibly use mindfulness within the 'professional story' (Healy, 2005). Knowledge creation within social work has traditionally relied 'on the assumption that systematically produced, "scientific", generalised and generalisable (propositional) knowledge provides the most solid foundations for practice' (Taylor, 2006: 4 in Trevithick, 2008: 1215). Contrary to this approach, these stories suggest that knowledge and use of mindfulness in social work is a contextual and relational process with social worker knowledge taking shape as their narrative of practice in the professional knowledge landscape unfolds. For some social workers, their own positioning within space, place and time in the professional context may create epistemological dilemmas around mindfulness that we understand narratively as 'secret' and 'sacred' stories (Clandinin & Connelly, 1996). These arise as they negotiate the 'professional story' of social work, within their professional knowledge landscape and what is considered to be appropriate knowledge for practice and practice decisions.

We believe that these stories show that the deeply contextual nature of the 'professional story' of social work indicates that the development of social work knowledge of mindfulness and embodied awareness requires new questions that take account of the complex environment in which social workers negotiate and undertake their practice. Moreover, it also highlights the need for new ways of understanding and relating to social workers' experience of reconciling mindfulness into their professional knowledge, context and identity within their 'professional story', and further exploration of the unique challenges and influences on the use of mindfulness in social work.

Acknowledgements

This manuscript has been supported by the CQUniversity **HEALTH CRN** www.cqu. edu.au/crn and the Australian Government's Collaborative Research Networks Program.

Disclosure statement

No potential conflict of interest was reported by the authors.

References

Bamberg, M (2006) 'Stories: big or small why do we care?', *Narrative Inquiry*, vol. 16, no. 1, pp. 139–147.

Bell, K (2012) 'Towards a post-conventional philosophical base for social work', *British Journal of Social Work*, vol. 42, pp. 408–423.

Berceli, D. & Napoli, M (2006) 'A proposal for mindfulness-based trauma prevention program for social work professionals', *Complementary Health Practice Review*, vol. 11, pp. 153–165.

Birnbaum, L. & Birnbaum, A (2008) 'Mindful social work: from theory to practice', *Journal of Religion and Spirituality In Social Work: Social Thought*, vol. 27, no. 1-2, pp. 87–104.

Bishop, SR, Lau, M, Shapiro, SS, Carlson, L, Anderson, ND, Carmody, J, Segal, ZV, Abbey, S, Speca, M, Velting, D. & Devins, G (2004) 'Mindfulness: a proposed operational definition', *Clinical Psychology: Science and Practice*, vol. 11, no. 3, pp. 230–241.

Bodhi, B (2011) 'What does mindfulness really mean? a canonical perspective', *Contemporary Buddhism*, vol. 12, no. 1, pp. 19–39.

Clandinin, DJ & Connelly, FM (1995) *Teachers' professional knowledge landscapes*, Teachers' College Press, New York.

Clandinin, DJ & Connelly, FM (1996) 'Teachers' professional knowledge landscapes: Teacher stories-stories of teachers-school stories-stories of schools', *Educational Researcher*, vol. 25, pp. 24–30.

Clandinin, DJ & Connelly, FM (2000) *Narrative Inquiry Experience and Story in Qualitative Research*, John Wiley & Sons Inc, San Francisco.

Coholic, D (2005) 'The helpfulness of spiritually influenced group work in developing self-awareness and self-esteem: a preliminary investigation', *The Scientific World Journal*, vol. 5, pp. 789–802.

Drury Hudson, J (1997) 'A model of professional knowledge for social work practice', *Australian Social Work*, vol. 50, no. 3, pp. 35–44.

Fenstermacher, GD (1994) 'The knower and the known: The nature of knowledge in research on teaching', *Review of Research in Education*, vol. 20, pp. 3–56.

Fook, J. (2002) *Social work: Critical theory and practice*, Sage Publications, London.

Fook, J, Ryan, M. & Hawkins, L (2000) *Professional Expertise: Practice, theory and Education for Working in Uncertainty*, Whiting and Birch, London.

Gause, R. & Coholic, D (2010) 'Mindfulness based practices as a holistic philosophy and method', *Currents: New Scholarship in the Human Services*, vol. 9, no. 2, http://currents.synergiesprairies.ca/currents/index.php/currents/article/view/42 (accessed 14 April 2013).

Grossman, P. & Van Dam, NT (2011) 'Mindfulness, by any other name . . . : Trials and tribulations of Sati in Western Psychology and science', *Contemporary Buddhism*, vol. 12, no. 1, pp. 219–239.

Hanh, T. N. (1976) *The Miracle of Mindfulness*, Beacon Press, Boston, MA.

Healy, K (2005) *Social Work Theories in Context: Creating Frameworks for Practice*, Palgrave MacMillan, Basingstoke.

Hick, SF (2008) 'My personal journey to mindfulness: implications for social work', *Reflections: Narratives of Professional Helping*, vol. 14, no. 2, pp. 16–23.

Hick, SF (2009) *Mindfulness and Social Work*, Lyceum Books, Inc, Chicago, IL.

Hick, SF & Furlotte, C (2009) 'Mindfulness and social justice approaches: Bridging the mind and society in social work practice', *Canadian Social Work*, vol. 26, no. 1, pp. 5–25.

Lee, M, Ng, S, Leung, P & Chan, C (2009) *Integrative Body-Mind-Spirit Social Work. An Empirically Based Approach to Assessment and Treatment*, Oxford University Press, New York.

Lynn, R (2010) 'Mindfulness in Social Work Education', *Social Work Education*, vol. 29, no. 3, pp. 289–304.

Lynn, R, Mensinga, J, Tinning, B & Lundman, K (2015) 'Is mindfulness value free? Tip toeing through the mindfield of mindfulness', in *Holistic Social Work Education in the 21st Century*, eds L Pyles & G Adam, Oxford University Press, New York, NY.

Mensinga, J (2010) *Quilting Professional Stories. A Gendered Experience of Choosing Social Work as a Career*, VDM Verlag Dr. Muller Aktiengesellschaft & Co. KG, Saarbrucken.

Mensinga, J (2011) 'The feeling of being a social worker: including yoga as an embodied practice in social work education', *Social Work Education*, vol. 30, no. 6, pp. 650–662.

Milton, I (2011) 'What does mindfulness really mean? Clarifying key terms and definitions: Part 1', *Psychotherapy in Australia*, vol. 17, no. 4, pp. 24–27.

Minor, HG. & Carlson, LE (2006) 'Evaluation of mindfulness-based stress reduction (MBSR) program for caregivers of children with chronic conditions', *Social Work in Health Care*, vol. 43, no. 1, pp. 91–109.

Ollerenshaw, JA. & Creswell, JW (2002) 'Narrative research: A comparison of two restorying data analysis approaches', *Qualitative Inquiry*, vol. 8, pp. 329.

Payne, M (1996) *What is Professional Social Work?* Venture Press, London.

Riessmann, CK (2007) *Narrative Methods for the Human Services*, Sage Publications, London.

Segal ZV, Hick SF. & Bien T (2010) *Mindfulness and the Therapeutic Relationship*, Guildford Publications, New York.

Taylor, C (2006) 'Narrating significant experience: Reflective accounts and the production of (self) knowledge', *British Journal of Social Work*, vol. 36, pp. 189–206.

Turner, K (2009) 'Mindfulness The present moment in clinical social work', *Clinical Social Work Journal*, vol. 37, no. 2, pp. 95–103.

Trevithick, P (2008) 'Revisiting the knowledge base of social work: A framework for practice', *British Journal of Social Work*, vol. 38, pp. 1212–1237.

Wallace, BA (2006) *The Attention Revolution*, Wisdom, Boston.

Wallace, BA (2011) *Minding Closely: The Four Applications of Mindfulness*, Snow Lion, New York.

Wallace, BA (2012) *Meditations for a Buddhist Sceptic: A Manifesto for the Mind Sciences and Contemplative Practice*, Columbia University Press, New York, NY.

Ya-Ling Chen, Barbara Rittner, Amy Manning and Rebekah Crofford

EARLY ONSET SCHIZOPHRENIA AND SCHOOL SOCIAL WORK

Schizophrenia, while most commonly adult onset, does occasionally occur in children and adolescents. Youths appropriately diagnosed with schizophrenia tend to have significantly lower school success and face more daily academic challenges which can be insurmountable. This article reviews prevalence rates, controversies associated with diagnosis, and school and social problems that youths with schizophrenia confront in the context of classifications, symptoms and course of childhood onset of schizophrenia. Implications for school social workers are discussed.

Overview of the disorder

In the USA, children with early onset schizophrenia and their families are burdened with both coping with the disorder and frustrations getting appropriate comprehensive services they need to manage the disorder. This is in contrast to many Western countries with more progressive, comprehensive and less fragmented health care where comprehensive services and treatment needs would be wholly or partly met by the state.

The general public and even many professionals view schizophrenia as a disorder with an onset in the late teens and early adulthood, although it has been recorded in childhood and early adolescence – with the caveat that it is a rare occurrence (Asarnow, 1994). Descriptions of various psychotic symptoms in children began to appear in the psychiatric literature at about the same time as descriptions of psychotic symptoms in adults (Asarnow & Asarnow, 1994). While schizophrenia is very rare in young children, there are documented incidents among children as young as 5 years of age (Russell *et al.*, 1989; Spencer *et al.*, 1992). Others argue that making a diagnosis of early onset psychosis or schizophrenia spectrum disorder is severely compromised by the difficulty of assessing thought disorder through middle latency because these children are resistant, and in many ways unable to discuss thought processes (Caplan, 1994).

There has been a delineation of three age-specific subgroups in schizophrenia: adult onset (AOS), early onset (EOS) and childhood onset (COS). AOS specifically refers to onset at or above the age of 20 years, EOS refers to onset before the 19th birthday while COS is specific to a diagnosis by age 13 years (Rhinewine *et al.*, 2005; Kumra *et al.*, 2009). In general, the 18th birthday is the most common cut-off age for EOS when it incorporates both EOS and COS (Rhinewine *et al.*, 2005; Burke *et al.*, 2008; Fulton *et al.*, 2008; Tang *et al.*, 2010). This paper focuses on those below age 18 with EOS, specifically those with a diagnosis of a schizophrenia spectrum disorder limited to schizophrenia, schizophreniform and schizoaffective disorder and excludes psychotic mood disorder or organic psychosis before their 18th birthday based on the International Statistical Classification of Diseases and Related Health Problems (ICD) or the Diagnostic and Statistical Manual of Mental Disorders (DSM) (Fagerlund *et al.*, 2006; Reichert *et al.*, 2008; Øie *et al.*, 2011).

Among the more common terms used to describe childhood presentation before age 18 of schizophrenia is early onset psychosis (EOP) (Thomsen, 1996; Fulton *et al.*, 2008), which encompasses schizophrenia, schizophreniform disorder, schizoaffective, psychotic mood disorders, psychosis not otherwise classified and organic psychosis (Sikich, 2008; Ledda *et al.*, 2009). Concerns are raised by the fact that increasingly more children are being treated with antipsychotics for non-psychotic diagnoses, leading to inflated assumptions about rates of EOP and what constitutes EOP. This position was reinforced by Olfson, Blanco, Liu, Moreno, and Laje (2006) who noted a sharp increase in physicians prescribing second-generation antipsychotic medications for disruptive behaviours associated with mood disorders and other disruptive behaviour diagnoses. Clearly youths on antipsychotic medications alone should not be considered indicative of EOP or EOS.

Associated behavioural and emotional characteristics in EOS

Early onset schizophrenia has always been subsumed under schizophrenia, although the definitions of childhood schizophrenia have been very variable (Asarnow *et al.*, 1994b; Cornblatt *et al.*, 1998). Historically there have been evolving representations and classifications of this disorder, resulting in a great deal of confusion. Before the 1970s, COS was categorized within the broader nosology of childhood psychosis, which puzzlingly included what is now referred to as autism spectrum disorder. The second edition of the Diagnostic and Statistical Manual of Mental Disorders (DSM-II) (American Psychiatric Association, 1968) required only psychotic speech and thoughts to make a diagnosis, but ironically failed to specify the current hallmark criteria of schizophrenia – hallucination and/or delusions. Not surprisingly, the DSM-II criteria resulted in problematic diagnostic overlaps with other psychotic disorders and within the pervasive developmental disorder spectrum, engendering the belief that autism was a form of psychotic disorder (McDonell & McClellan, 2007). The proposed revisions for the DSM-III included attempts to resolve the diagnostic confusion differentiating EOS, infantile autism and pervasive developmental disorders by creating distinct diagnostic criteria for each (Rutter, 1972). Beginning with the DSM-III and in the current schematics for schizophrenia in both the ICD and the DSM, schizophrenia requires psychotic symptoms such as presentation of bizarre delusions and presence of hallucinations. They do not, however, delineate differential aspects for COS, EOS and

AOS (McDonell & McClellan, 2007). In the development of the DSM-V, the American Psychiatric Association did not provide specific symptoms for EOS but did note that earlier onset predicts a poorer outcome (APA, 2014).

Onset patterns in youth with schizophrenia

The literature suggests that any psychiatric diagnoses in children should be considered with suspicion. As Kim-Cohen *et al.* (2003) correctly observed, over diagnose psychiatric disorders are common in children, and in their longitudinal study, EOS seemed to be especially unreliable. Furthermore, discussions about severe childhood responses to adverse childhood events, extreme poverty, neglect and trauma appear implicated in both the onset of schizophrenia and the severity of the symptoms, but there has been little systematic research in recent years supporting these as contributing factors (Caton *et al.*, 1998). Most recently, DeRosse *et al.* (2014) attempted to assess the correlation between trauma and abuse histories with increased risk for psychotic symptoms in hospitalized patients compared to general population controls, but found the differences were not statically significant.

In reality, little is known about its aetiology or long-term disease process. Prevalence rates for EOS show it is more common in males (Green *et al.*, 1992; Schothorst *et al.*, 2006). Chronic or insidious onset appears more common in males under the age of 12, and acute onset is more common in females approaching adulthood (Green *et al.*, 1992; Thomsen, 1996; Eggers & Bunk, 1997). In the premorbid period, only some youths are entirely behaviourally and cognitively normal prior to the onset of illness; and it is during this phase that both positive symptoms of hallucinations and delusions as well as the negative withdrawal and introversion symptoms emerge (Hollis, 2003; McClellan *et al.* 2003; Schothorst *et al.*, 2006; Wozniak *et al.*, 2008; Meng *et al.*, 2009).

Equally uncertain are possible premorbid and comorbid conditions associated with an increased probability for EOS, including the role of attention-deficit hyperactive disorder and development of psychosis in youths with family histories of schizophrenia, but findings were inconclusive (Keshavan *et al.*, 2003). Many youths with schizophrenia present with depressive symptoms prior to their transition to psychotic symptoms, and there is apparent continuity in severity of depressive symptoms over the developmental course of the illness (Myles-Worsley *et al.*, 2007). A recent study found links to severe depression, negative schizophrenia symptoms and higher rates of suicide attempts, especially with comorbid alcohol use in males with EOS (Romm *et al.*, 2010). Models have been developed to examine the role of cortical activity in post-traumatic stress and attention-deficit disorders as a trigger for EOS, but findings suggest that they are discrete comorbid disorders rather than predictive or part of a spectrum (Rowe *et al.*, 2004). Additional research on phenomenological, cognitive, neuroimaging and genetic data indicates that cognitive and neurobiological abnormalities are similar in EOS and AOS (Kumra & Schulz, 2008). However, course variability in COS appears greater than is observed in AOS, and it appears that COS results in more severe symptoms and consequences over time (Eggers *et al.*, 2000).

There has been some exploration of genetic vulnerability in EOS (Ota *et al.*, 2010), suggesting greater genetic predisposition and susceptibility in families with histories of EOS and COS. Neurodevelopmental abnormalities are generally accepted as part of the presentation of schizophrenia, although much of this work has been done on adults using retrospective data (Hata, *et al.*, 2003). Premorbid and prodromal periods show abnormalities in early brain development; eventually these abnormalities lead to failures to attain expected developmental milestones as well as functional decline (Kumra & Schulz, 2008; Ota *et al.*, 2010).

It is also worth noting that some studies are beginning to suggest that these abnormalities may be associated with the long-term side effects of antipsychotics rather than a distinct disease process or genetically caused abnormalities (Whitaker, 2004). Regardless of the cause, abnormalities in white matter, cortical grey matter or structural aberration of the brains have been observed in youths with EOS (Sowell *et al.*, 2000; Burke *et al.*, 2008; Penttilä *et al.*, 2008; Kumra *et al.*, 2009; Tang *et al.*, 2010).

Antipsychotic medication and youths with EOS

There is controversy about the benefits of antipsychotic medication; and findings on subjective experiences would challenge the assumptions of improved cognition, given that most users reporting on a consumer website indicated they experienced sedation and "cognitive and emotional flattening" (Moncreiff *et al.*, 2009, p. 102; Marquis *et al.* 2011). Indifference, depression, sexual impairment and mental restlessness were reported as the most common impact of the medications (Moncreiff *et al.*, 2009).

Given the impact on possible cognitive functioning of typical and atypical antipsychotics and known patterns of withdrawal and depression as part of prodromal symptoms in EOS, assumptions about overall intellectual functioning and learning disabilities in this population should be considered with caution. However, current research suggests that youths with EOS test below the standardized IQ normative mean, have greater delays in verbal, visual and working memory and display fewer adaptive life skills; although it is difficult to determine if this is due to the disorder or the effects of medications (Asarnow *et al.*, 1994a; Fagerlund *et al.*, 2006; Kester *et al.*, 2006; Walder *et al.*, 2006; Puig *et al.*, 2012). Regardless, cognitive deficits exist across multiple domains, suggesting widespread brain dysfunction in EOS youths (Rhinewine *et al.*, 2005).

Long-term outcome for youth with EOS

Children with early onset schizophrenia confront numerous problems which compromise their familial, academic and social functioning and create wide variances in outcomes as they mature into adulthood (Jarbin *et al.*, 2003; Schothorst *et al.*, 2006; Reichert *et al.*, 2008). Many have histories of other co-morbid psychiatric illnesses, social skills deficits, speech and language delays and motor developmental problems as well as educational failures (Schothorst *et al.*, 2006; Fulton *et al.*, 2008).

Long-term outcomes vary according to the targeted end stage dimension evaluated. One study on psychotic symptomology showed 60% experienced moderate, 20% showed minimal and 17% showed no significant improvement in symptoms over time (Green *et al.*, 1992). Based on global adjustment and psychosocial functioning, another study indicated that 45% showed deteriorating course or minimal improvement, 28% showed moderate improvement and 28% showed good improvement (Asarnow & Tompson, 1999). A 13-year follow-up study conducted in Germany showed 22% of former patients with EOS still experience acute schizophrenic symptoms at follow-up, and 77% were still in outpatient treatment (Reichert *et al.*, 2008).

School outcomes of those with EOS

Children with EOS and COS receive services for severe emotional disturbances (SEDs) and are considered eligible for comprehensive programmes under the latest Individuals with Disability Educational Act (IDEA, 2004 Nos. 108-77). Over six million students aged 6 through 21were receiving special needs services through IDEA, representing 9.1% of school-age children; and, according to the latest available congressional report (U.S. Department of Education, 2008), of those, 7.5% were identified as having emotional problems. Students with EOS and COS as well as other mental health problems often experience multiple school placements unrelated to parental changes in residence. Malmgren and Meisel (2004) noted that children identified as SED had higher rates of school replacements with 72% attending more than one school, even after being placed in special education and, in aggregate, have among the highest dropout rate (44.9%) of all students of ages 14−21 served under IDEA.

In general, children with histories of SED are among the lowest performing special needs students, especially when they have additional comorbid learning and psychiatric conditions (Anderson *et al.*, 2001). On standard tests, adults with schizophrenia often scored well below the 50th percentile in 4th, 8th and 11th grades, and evidenced linear decline in language scores over time in a longitudinal study (Fuller *et al.*, 2002). Interestingly, this study supported Cannon's earlier finding that academic scores at grades 4 and 8 were not below average but dropped significantly between grades 8 and 11, suggestive of emerging cognitive deficits in students with COS and EOS either as part of the disease process, comorbid depression or medication effects (Cannon *et al.*, 1999). In general, children with SED have comprehensive deficits in reading, spelling and arithmetic (Hooper *et al.*, 2010), but those with EOS consistently show poorer academic achievement, lower standardized math and verbal scores, and more disciplinary and social problems (Anderson *et al.*, 2001; Schothorst, *et al.*, 2006).

Finally, problematic school behaviours associated with poor impulse control (such as disruptive behaviours, aggression and disrespectful behaviours) are known symptoms in these populations (COS and EOS) and create adverse consequences, particularly in schools with "zero tolerance" policies for non-compliant behaviours (Malmgren & Meisel, 2004; Algozzine *et al.*, 2008). Many students with COS and EOS struggle with remaining in their seats, avoiding being distracted, processing information, memorizing and taking tests, and, not surprisingly, find school frustrating and depressing and suffer from the severe consequences of multiple suspensions and expulsions (Myles-Worsley *et al.*, 2007).

Services required but not provided

Between 1995 and 2004 in the USA, the total number of students aged 6 through 21 receiving special educational services increased from 5.1 million to more than 6.1 million in the 50 states and DC. Of those, 7.9% were youths with SED in 2004 with an estimated annual cost of $12,639 per student for appropriate additional educational services (U.S. Department of Education, 2003). Clearly, given the high dropout rate, educational needs are not being met for these students. Among contributing factors is that these students often shift into special settings 60% of the day both within school settings and in a variety of specialized day-treatment school and inpatient settings. As demands for services escalate, resources to provide those services become stretched in schools with limited budgets, particularly in light of resistance to higher school taxes in communities struggling to match resources to a wide variety of required services.

Ideally, individual educational plans (IEPs) for this population should incorporate instructional goals coupled with social skills training, but rarely do. Positive pro-social peer interactions are essential in youths with EOS for development of social networks and to counteract experiences of being alone and isolated after hospitalizations or residential treatment, especially given medication side effects (Puig *et al.*, 2012; Remschmidt & Theisen, 2012). In addition, coordinating with ancillary services (occupational, rehabilitative, mental health and health) is implicit in successful outcomes. Many psycho-skills training elements fall under occupational therapy skills, including learning how to have conversations (Liberman *et al.*, 1998).

Case example

A 14-year-old student had been diagnosed with EOS beginning at age 11years and had five psychiatric hospitalizations in 3 years. He has a history of poor academic achievement, agitation, fighting with peers and teachers, as well as depression and anxiety. He has few friends and is often the object of bullies who tease and taunt him. In the last week he has been heard arguing with voices and engages in repetitive and ritualized behaviours disruptive to other students. He was suspended for smoking on campus twice in the last month. He refuses his medication because it is "poison". He tells the school social worker that smoking quiets the voices and then admits in a confidential tone that intergalactic aliens are coming to return him to the galaxy where he was born. His physician wants to hospitalize him, and both the student and parents are resistant. The parents are aware of his "ideas" and report that, every time the doorbell rings, the youth hides in the closet or under the bed. The impoverished parents support their child in refusing hospitalization and medications in part because of the cost.

Roles for school social workers with youth with EOS

Interpreting the diagnosis and assessing medication impact

There is often an assumption that families fully understand their children's diagnoses and that, with the availability of Internet resources, a great deal of information is accessible to them. However, entering "childhood schizophrenia" into a common search engine results in over 30 pages of links. Often distressed families struggle to understand available materials, much of which is contradictory. School social workers, in the absence of another advocate, can help families decide whether they feel diagnoses are accurate, what they can expect if they are and what the role of medications are in treating the symptoms of delusions and hallucinations. Social workers should be cognizant of off-label use of antipsychotic medication and the impact of diagnostic labels based solely on types of medication rather than symptom presentation. Stafford (2006) asked whether there should be better federal oversight by the Food and Drug Administration in the USA of the wide use of off-label antipsychotic medications, especially with children, for reasons other than psychotic symptoms (most often for depression and behavioural problems), precisely because of serious side effects and unintended labelling of these children as having psychotic disorders.

In the case study, a school social worker could help by providing some basic information to the family (including useful links that follow frequently asked questions [FAQs]) about the diagnosis. This includes helping them understand symptoms in the context of fluctuating presentation and levels of stress. Management of delusions and hallucinations without conflicts about "reality" is critical because those delusions and hallucinations are both "real" experiences to the youth. There are also simulations that can help the family members understand the experience of auditory hallucinations and why the person often engages in conversations with those hallucinations. This can foster a better understanding of symptoms and their impact on behaviours.

School social workers can encourage youth and their caregivers to keep medication logs to track ancillary information about adherence and non-adherence against symptom presentation and side effects and to serve as potentially powerful tools for youth and caregivers to use when consulting with prescribers about possible nuanced medication regimens. More critically, if all medications are listed, including herbal and other over-the-counter medications along with those prescribed by medical professionals, negative side effects and toxic drug interactions can be identified early to prevent potential life-threatening consequences. As part of casework services, school social workers can encourage families to work with trusted pharmacists or health care providers to balance the need for medication against potential side effects that can lead to fatalities because of cardiovascular, pulmonary, neurological, endocrine and gastrointestinal complications (Spencer et al., 1992; Hrdlicka & Dudova, 2007; Kumra et al., 2008; Haas et al., 2009; Kryzhanovskaya et al., 2009; Robb et al., 2010; Levine & Ruha 2012). It is worth noting that Whitaker (2004) and others (Spina et al., 2002) have expressed concerns about the toxicity of antipsychotics, and Whitaker, in particular, is advocating for the use of less or no medications at the same time as families often report that physicians and other health care professionals tend to add additional medications in attempts to manage thought and behavioural problems (The Medicated Child, Introduction, 2009).

School social worker strategies

School social workers often are the point persons coordinating services for children with EOS within school systems and bear responsibilities for tracking down resources, evaluating outcomes and providing feedback for stakeholders working with children with early onset schizophrenia. There is very little in the empirical literature to support alternative approaches to treating EOS, although youths, like their adult counterparts, seek alternatives to medication approaches. School social workers would benefit from exploring with youths with EOS and their caregivers what alternative approaches they have researched on the Internet including animal-assisted therapy, music therapy, Chinese herbal therapies and so on. A frank and non-judgmental discussion about these approaches with the youth and their caregivers as alternatives to medications or reduced levels of medication could reduce the potential for covert alternative treatments and might be incorporated into the IEP (Complementary Schizophrenia Treatments, n.d.). Consideration of cognitive-behavioural approaches to manage symptoms, using music and other auditory approaches to block intrusive voice commands and commentaries, may be more effective than increased levels of medication or traditional disciplinary actions (such as suspensions) in reducing behaviour problems associated with delusions and hallucinations. Some families have also tried possible dietary adjustments or vitamins and supplements to manage symptoms that may also help students adjust better to classroom settings.

Helping to manage financial and the social services

There are enormous financial, social, emotional and physical stressors on family members adjusting to a diagnosis of schizophrenia, including learning how to manage the symptoms of the disorder at home and in school and social settings, particularly in the USA where insurance coverage can be problematic and subject to significant limitations, exclusions and discontinuances. School social workers can reduce some of the initial stress by providing contact information on possible community-based resources. While ideally the coordination of resources should be part of the initial diagnosis and certainly part of hospital discharge planning, not all children with EOS are hospitalized and not all mental health clinics provide families with supportive services. These support systems particularly help caregivers navigate the frustration of completing the paperwork needed to obtain services through various educational, medical and mental health systems.

Linking caregivers to support networks also often provides information about strategies for successfully processing insurance claims and possible appeals on denial of services. Peers in these networks frequently can direct families to legal resources which they might need in appeals processes. They can provide guidance about how best to complete applications for disability benefits, determining rights to family leave, assessing the merits of local service delivery systems and resources, and developing plans for respite services. Many of them are knowledgeable about medication issues and locating prescription providers within insurance plans and networks. In the case example, this might diminish some of the family's financial concerns regarding the cost of medication and the challenges in hospitalization.

School social workers are often relied upon to find creative ways to help family members function optimally at home and school. Helping the family in the case example learn to de-escalate symptom exacerbation may also reduce the need for hospitalization by helping stabilize behaviours and may also reduce the need for higher levels of medications. In addition, social workers can connect the family to local mental health support groups. These support groups can work with the family to tailor strategies to manage symptoms as well as provide venues for recreation and socialization. Increased socialization may diminish isolation – especially if it also connects the family to a supportive network able to provide respite services.

Because of the rarity of the diagnosis, it is important for the social worker to develop an FAQ for the teachers and aides to help them understand what EOS is and is not, what impact the diagnosis might have on processing curricular content, what medications the youth is on and the impact of medications on learning, what the signs are of decompensation and escalation of psychotic symptoms and possible early interventions which might delimit it. It is critical that teachers and aides learn to differentiate behaviours associated with the disorder from other age appropriate or inappropriate acting out when making disciplinary decisions (Malmgren & Meisel, 2004; Algozzine *et al.*, 2008).

In the case example, the social worker could locate practitioners who use cognitive-behavioural techniques with people with schizophrenia as an enhancement to or alternative to medications to promote better reality testing and to help regulate behaviours that contribute to being taunted and bullied. With open communication lines, the social worker could coordinate treatment strategies with family members, teachers and aides who focus on reduction of reactivity to voices – a source of ongoing classroom problems (see Christodoulides *et al.*, 2008).

Managing hospitalizations

Sudden inpatient hospitalizations can occur to manage acute exacerbation of psychotic symptoms (Kumra & Schulz, 2008). The school social worker can work with teachers to coordinate educational resources and assignments as appropriate during the hospitalization. The social worker should coordinate the transfer of relevant information between systems both during the hospitalization and during discharge planning. Managing return to school following hospital discharge or other therapeutic placements should include ensuring treatment, and medication protocols are incorporated into the development of an IEP or amended IEP as part of transitional services between the therapeutic setting and the school. It is a role that may well fall to the school social worker. When the youth is ready to return to school, the school social worker can provide supportive assistance with integration back into the routine of school.

Involvement in the individualized educational plan

School social workers have a central role in ensuring that IEP's incorporate family input and that needed services are identified, especially at the point of re-entry to school. This is especially important since IEP teams may become quite formulaic about the components of plans based on more commonly seen learning disabilities. Because of the complexity of EOS, the IEP should have feedback loops and tracking mechanisms across multiple providers (caregivers, youth, teachers, school nurses, outpatient and psychiatric services, occupational and rehabilitation therapists, mental health providers, etc.) so that plans are comprehensive enough to ensure delivery of needed primary and ancillary services. Furthermore, these plans should include schematics about how team members communicate with each other and who is key worker for which elements in the plan (medication, symptom management, de-escalation of symptoms, etc.). This is an effective mechanism to identify problems early, develop solutions across appropriate systems and monitor outcomes against IEP goals, suggesting changes as indicated. This becomes especially critical when there are changes in school placement either because of reassignments within school systems, hospital admissions or transfer to residential placements so that there is continuity of services.

In the case example, the IEP should address the use of tobacco to manage psychotic symptoms, both because it is illegal and because it violates school rules resulting in disciplinary actions. Including cognitive-behavioural mindfulness techniques may delimit some of the anxiety and depressive symptoms, thereby reducing psychotic symptoms. These techniques are especially useful as a healthy alternative to tobacco when they are adapted to youths with EOS who smoke (Cown & Reibel, 2010). Involving the youths in how these techniques can be implemented during the school day and at home may be one way to encourage compliance with mindfulness techniques.

School social workers can work with youths about how much information to share with peers and how to manage bullying and other negative peer encounters. Many youths who are diagnosed with EOS find that acute exacerbation of symptoms compounds their problems, especially in the context of side effects of medications and delusional and psychotic symptoms. To address these issues, some school social workers develop peer support groups, if possible, for youths with SEDs. Depending on the size of the student body, however, these groups may focus either on supports for students with disabilities, students with recent psychiatric hospitalizations or more generalized social skills groups which provide coaching on appropriate and positive peer interactions.

School social workers should help school personnel consider possible responses to acting out associated with psychotic symptoms that differ from customary disciplinary responses (suspensions and expulsions) in order to adopt more appropriate and reasonable accommodations (Francis *et al.*, 2012). School social workers can provide teachers, staff and administrators with sufficient knowledge about techniques to de-escalate psychotic reactivity, especially those that re-enforce reality testing and self-calming behaviours.

Conclusion

Youths with EOS are a rare population. School social workers may never encounter a student diagnosed with EOS during their career, and face the challenge of finding experienced school social worker peers as a mentor and resource. This suggests the importance of professional learning networks (PLNs) in general but especially when working with a very complex and difficult problems, such as rare conditions such as EOS, that require complex and well-coordinated case plans. Access to PLNs, many of which are now web based, can provide both knowledge and strategies that may not be regionally available to an individual social worker. These PLNs are often transdisciplinary with professionals working in a variety of fields, including education, mental health, medicine, occupational and rehabilitation therapy, and in communities. There are a variety of means of access to them, from connecting through national organizations such as the National Alliance for Mental Illness, contacting practitioners who have made podcasts or given presentations, to joining Twitter® discussions or following blogs. These resources often provide access to webinars and conferences where a social worker can directly discuss the issues with more experienced practitioners and find creative solutions. This can lead to enhanced e-learning partnerships. Many digital resources are tailored to schizophrenia and are followed by professionals who work with this population and can serve as invaluable resources to school social workers and families. Finally, contacting authors of papers that the practitioner has found invaluable may lead to a mentor or an expanded network of other practitioners with more experience.

References

Algozzine, K., Christian, C., Marr, M. B., McClanahan, T. & White, R. (2008) 'Demography of problem behavior in elementary schools', *Exceptionality*, vol. 16, no. 2, pp. 93–104. doi:10.1080/09362830801981369.

Anderson, J. A., Kutash, K. & Duchnowski, A. J. (2001) 'A comparison of the academic progress of students with EBD and students with LD', *Journal of Emotional and Behavioral Disorders*, vol. 9, no. 2, pp. 106–115. doi:10.1177/106342660100900205.

Asarnow, J. R. (1994) 'Childhood-Onset Schizophrenia', *Journal of Child Psychology And Psychiatry, And Allied Disciplines*, vol. 35, no. 8, pp. 1345–1371. doi:10.1111/j.1469-7610.1994.tb01280.x.

Asarnow, R. F., Asamen, J., Granholm, E. & Sherman, T. (1994) 'Cognitive/neuropsychological studies of children with a schizophrenic disorder', *Schizophrenia Bulletin*, vol. 20, no. 4, pp. 647–669. doi:10.1093/schbul/20.4.647.

Asarnow, J. R., Tompson, M. C. & Goldstein, M. J. (1994) 'Childhood-onset schizophrenia: a followup study', *Schizophrenia Bulletin*, vol. 20, no. 4, pp. 599–617. doi:10.1093/schbul/20.4.599.

Asarnow, R. F. & Asarnow, J. R. (1994) 'Childhood-onset schizophrenia: editors' introduction', *Schizophrenia Bulletin*, vol. 20, no. 4, pp. 591–597. doi:10.1093/schbul/20.4.591.

Asarnow, R. J. & Tompson, M. C. (1999) 'Childhood-onset schizophrenia: a follow-up study', *European Child & Adolescent Psychiatry*, vol. 8, no. S1, pp. S9–S12. doi:10.1007/PL00010685.

American Psychiatric Association. (1968) *Diagnostic and Statistical Manual of Mental Disorders (DSM-II)*. 2nd ed. American Psychiatric Association, Washington, DC.

American Psychiatric Association. (2014) *Diagnostic and Statistical Manual of Mental Disorders (DSM-V)*. 5th ed. American Psychiatric Association, Washington, DC. Retrieved from http://www.dsm5.org

Burke, L., Androutsos, C., Jogia, J., Byrne, P. & Frangou, S. (2008) 'The Maudsley Early Onset Schizophrenia Study: the effect of age of onset and illness duration on fronto-parietal gray matter', *European Psychiatry*, vol. 23, no. 4, pp. 233–236. doi:10.1016/j.eurpsy.2008.03.007.

Cannon, M., Jones, P., Huttunen, M. O., Tanskanen, A., Huttunen, T., Rabe-Hesketh, S. & Murray, R. M. (1999) 'School performance in Finnish children and later development of schizophrenia', *Archives of General Psychiatry*, vol. 56, no. 5, pp. 457–463. doi:10.1001/archpsyc.56.5.457.

Caplan, R. (1994) 'Communication deficits in childhood schizophrenia spectrum disorders', *Schizophrenia Bulletin*, vol. 20, no. 4, pp. 671–683. doi:10.1093/schbul/20.4.671.

Caton, C. M., Cournos, F., Felix, A. & Wyatt, R. J. (1998) 'Childhood experiences and current adjustment of offspring of indigent patients with schizophrenia', *Psychiatric Services*, vol. 49, no. 1, pp. 86–90. doi:10.1176/ps.49.1.86.

Christodoulides, T., Dudley, R., Brown, S., Turkington, D. & Beck, A. T. (2008) 'Cognitive behaviour therapy in patients with schizophrenia who are not prescribed antipsychotic medication: a case series', *Psychology and Psychotherapy: Theory, Research And Practice*, vol. 81, no. 2, pp. 199–207. doi:10.1348/147608308X278295.

Complementary Schizophrenia Treatments. (n.d.). Retrieved from http://www.schizophrenia.com/treatments.php

Cornblatt, B., Obuchowski, M., Schnur, D. & O'Brien, J. D. (1998) 'Hillside study of risk and early detection in schizophrenia', *British Journal of Psychiatry*, vol. 172, no. (Suppl 33), pp. 26–32.

Cown, D. & Reibel, D. (2010) 'Mindfulness and mindfulness-based stress reduction', in *Integrative Psychiatry*, eds D. A. Monti & B. D. Beitman, Oxford University Press, New York, pp. 289–338.

DeRosse, P., Nitzburg, G. C., Kompancaril, B. & Malhotra, A. K. (2014) 'The relation between childhood maltreatment and psychosis in patients with schizophrenia and non-psychiatric controls', *Schizophrenia Research*, vol. 155, no. 1–3, pp. 66–71. doi:10.1016/j.schres.2014.03.009.

Eggers, C. & Bunk, D. (1997) 'The long-term course of childhood-onset schizophrenia: A 42-year followup', *Schizophrenia Bulletin*, vol. 23, no. 1, pp. 105–117. doi:10.1093/schbul/23.1.105.

Eggers, C., Bunk, D. & Krause, D. (2000) 'Schizophrenia with onset before the age of eleven: clinical characteristics of onset and course', *Journal of Autism and Developmental Disorders*, vol. 30, no. 1, pp. 29–38. doi:10.1023/A:1005408010797.

Fagerlund, B., Pagsberg, A. K. & Hemmingsen, R. P. (2006) 'Cognitive deficits and levels of IQ in adolescent onset schizophrenia and other psychotic disorders?', *Schizophrenia Research*, vol. 85, no. 1-3, pp. 30–39. doi:10.1016/j.schres.2006.03.004.

Francis, S., Ebesutani, C. & Chorpita, B. (2012) 'Differences in levels of functional impairment and rates of serious emotional disturbance between youth with internalizing and externalizing disorders when using the CAFAS or GAF to assess functional impairment', *Journal of Emotional & Behavioral Disorders*, vol. 20, no. 4, pp. 226–240. doi:10.1177/1063426610387607.

Fuller, R., Nopoulos, P., Arndt, S., O'leary, D., Ho, B. -C. & Andreasen, N. C. (2002) 'Longitudinal assessment of premorbid cognitive functioning in patients with schizophrenia through examination of standardized scholastic test performance', *The American Journal of Psychiatry*, vol. 159, no. 7, pp. 1183–1189. doi:10.1176/appi.ajp.159.7.1183.

Fulton, K., Short, M., Harvey-Smith, D., Rushe, T. M. & Mulholland, C. (2008) 'The Northern Ireland Early Onset Psychosis Study: phenomenology and co-morbidity in the first 25 cases', *Child Care in Practice*, vol. 14, no. 2, pp. 207–216. doi:10.1080/13575270701868884.

Green, W. H., Padron-Gayol, M., Hardesty, A. S. & Bassiri, M. (1992) 'Schizophrenia with childhood onset: a phenomenological study of 38 cases', *Journal of the American Academy of Child & Adolescent Psychiatry*, vol. 31, no. 5, pp. 968–976. doi:10.1097/00004583-199209000-00027.

Haas, M., Unis, A. S., Armenteros, J., Copenhaver, M. D., Quiroz, J. A. & Kushner, S. F. (2009) 'A 6-week, randomized, double-blind, placebo-controlled study of the efficacy and safety of risperidone in adolescents with schizophrenia', *Journal of Child and Adolescent Psychopharmacology*, vol. 19, no. 6, pp. 611–621. doi:10.1089/cap.2008.0144.

Hata, K., Iida, J., Iwasaka, H., Negoro, H. I., Ueda, F. & Kishimoto, T. (2003) 'Minor physical anomalies in childhood and adolescent onset schizophrenia', *Psychiatry and Clinical Neurosciences*, vol. 57, no. 1, pp. 17–21. doi:10.1046/j.1440-1819.2003.01074.x.

Hollis, C. (2003) 'Developmental precursors of child- and adolescent-onset schizophrenia and affective psychoses: Diagnostic specificity and continuity with symptom dimensions', *British Journal of Psychiatry*, vol. 182, no. 1, pp. 37–44. doi:10.1192/bjp.182.1.37.

Hooper, S. R., Giuliano, A. J., Youngstrom, E. A., Breiger, D., Sikich, L., Frazier, J. A., Findling, R. L., McClellan, J., Hamer, R. M., Vitiello, B. & Lieberman, J. A. (2010) 'Neurocognition in early-onset schizophrenia and schizoaffective disorders', *Journal of the American Academy of Child & Adolescent Psychiatry*, vol. 49, no. 1, pp. 52–60.

Hrdlicka, M. & Dudova, I. (2007) 'Risperidone in adolescent schizophrenic psychoses: a retrospective study', *International Journal of Psychiatry in Clinical Practice*, vol. 11, no. 4, pp. 273–278. doi:10.1080/13651500701246054.

Individuals with Disabilities Education Improvement Act. (2004) 'Building the legacy: IDEA 2004'. 118 STAT. 2781-2784. Retrieved October 27, 2014, from http://idea.ed.gov/explore/view/p/%2Croot%2Cstatute%2C

Jarbin, H., Ott, Y. & von Knorring, A. L. (2003) 'Adult outcome of social function in adolescent-onset schizophrenia and affective psychosis', *Journal of the American Academy of Child & Adolescent Psychiatry*, vol. 42, no. 2, pp. 176–183. doi:10.1097/00004583-200302000-00011.

Keshavan, M. S., Sujata, M., Mehra, A., Montrose, D. M. & Sweeney, J. A. (2003) 'Psychosis proneness and ADHD in young relatives of schizophrenia patients', *Schizophrenia Research*, vol. 59, no. 1, pp. 85–92. doi:10.1016/S0920-9964(01)00400-5.

Kester, H. M., Sevy, S., Yechiam, E., Burdick, K. E., Cervellione, K. L. & Kumra, S. (2006) 'Decision-making impairments in adolescents with early-onset schizophrenia', *Schizophrenia Research*, vol. 85, nos. 1–3, pp. 113–123. doi:10.1016/j.schres.2006.02.028.

Kim-Cohen, J., Caspi, A., Moffitt, T. E., Harrington, H., Milne, B. J. & Poulton, R. (2003) 'Prior juvenile diagnoses in adults with mental disorder', *Archives of General Psychiatry*, vol. 60, no. 7, pp. 709–717. doi:10.1001/archpsyc.60.7.709.

Kryzhanovskaya, L., Schulz, S. C., McDougle, C., Frazier, J., Dittmann, R., Robertson-Plouch, C., Bauer, T., Xu, W., Wang, W., Carlson, J. & Tohen, M. (2009) 'Olanzapine versus placebo in adolescents with schizophrenia: A 6-week, randomized, double-blind, placebo-controlled trial', *Journal of the American Academy of Child & Adolescent Psychiatry*, vol. 48, no. 1, pp. 60–70. doi:10.1097/CHI.0b013e3181900404.

Kumra, S., Asarnow, R., Grace, A., Keshavan, M., McClellan, J., Sikich, L. & Wagner, A. (2009) 'From bench to bedside: Translating new research from genetics and neuroimaging into treatment development for early-onset schizophrenia', *Early Intervention in Psychiatry*, vol. 3, no. 4, pp. 243–258. doi:10.1111/j.1751-7893.2009.00142.x.

Kumra, S., Kranzler, H., Gerbino-Rosen, G., Kester, H. M., DeThomas, C., Kafantaris, V., Correll, C. U. & Kane, J. M. (2008) 'Clozapine and "high-dose" olanzapine in refractory early-onset schizophrenia: A 12-week randomized and double-blind comparison', *Biological Psychiatry*, vol. 63, no. 5, pp. 524–529. doi:10.1016/j.biopsych.2007.04.043.

Kumra, S. & Schulz, S. C. (2008) 'Research progress in early-onset schizophrenia', *Schizophrenia Bulletin*, vol. 34, no. 1, pp. 15–17. doi:10.1093/schbul/sbm123.

Ledda, M. G., Fratta, A. L., Pintor, M., Zuddas, A. & Cianchetti, C. (2009) 'Early-onset psychoses: Comparison of clinical features and adult outcome in 3 diagnostic groups', *Child Psychiatry and Human Development*, vol. 40, no. 3, pp. 421–437.

Levine, M. & Ruha, A. M. (2012) 'Overdose of atypical antipsychotics: clinical presentation, mechanisms of toxicity and management', *CNS Drugs*, vol. 26, no. 7, pp. 601–611. Retrieved from www.ncbi.nlm.nih.gov/pubmed/22668123

Liberman, R. P., Wallace, C. J., Blackwell, G., Kopelowicz, A., Vaccaro, J. V. & Mintz, J. (1998) 'Skills training versus psychosocial occupational therapy for persons with persistent schizophrenia', *American Journal of Psychiatry*, vol. 155, pp. 1087–1091.

Malmgren, K. & Meisel, S. (2004) 'Examining the link between child maltreatment and delinquency for youth with emotional and behavioral disorders', *Child Welfare*, vol. 83, no. 2, pp. 175–188.

Marquis, K., Comery, T., Jow, F., Navarra, R., Grauer, S., Pulicicchio, C., Kelley, C., Brennan, J., Roncarati, R., Scali, C., Haydar, S., Ghiron, C., Terstappen, G. & Dunlop, J. (2011) 'Preclinical assessment of an adjunctive treatment approach for cognitive impairment associated with schizophrenia using the alpha7 nicotinic acetylcholine receptor agonist WYE-103914/SEN34625', *Psychopharmacology*, vol. 218, no. 4, pp. 635–647. doi:10.1007/s00213-011-2357-6.

McClellan, J., Breiger, M., McCurry, C. & Hlastala, S. A. (2003) 'Premorbid functioning in early-onset psychotic disorders', *Journal of the American Academy of Child & Adolescent Psychiatry*, vol. 42, no. 6, pp. 666–672.

McDonell, M. G. & McClellan, J. M. (2007) 'Early-onset schizophrenia', in *Assessment of Childhood Disorders*, eds E. J. Mash & R. A. Barkley. 4th ed. Guilford Press, New York, pp. 526–550.

Meng, H., Graf Schimmelmann, B., Koch, E., Bailey, B., Parzer, P., Günter, M., Mohler, B., Kunz, N., Schulte-Markwort, M., Felder, W., Zollinger, R., Bürgin, D. & Resch, F. (2009) 'Basic symptoms in the general population and in psychotic and non-psychotic psychiatric adolescents', *Schizophrenia Research*, vol. 111, no. 1-3, pp. 32–38.

Moncreiff, J., Cohwn, D. & Mason, J. P. (2009) 'The subjective experience of taking antipsychotic medication: a content analysis of Internet data', *Acta Psychiatry Scandanavia*, vol. 120, pp. 102–111. doi:10.1111/j.1600-0447.2009.01356.x.

Myles-Worsley, M., Weaver, S. & Blailes, F. (2007) 'Comorbid depressive symptoms in the developmental course of adolescent-onset psychosis', *Early Intervention in Psychiatry*, vol. 1, no. 2, pp. 183–190.

Olfson, M., Blanco, C., Liu, L., Moreno, C. & Laje, G. (2006) 'National trends in the outpatient treatment of children and adolescents with antipsychotic drugs', *Archives of General Psychiatry*, vol. 63, no. 6, pp. 679–685.

Øie, M., Sundet, K. & Ueland, T. (2011) 'Neurocognition and functional outcome in early-onset schizophrenia and attention-deficit/hyperactivity disorder: A 13-year follow-up', *Neuropsychology*, vol. 25, no. 1, pp. 25–35. doi:10.1037/a0020855.

Ota, V. K., Belangero, S. I., Gadelha, A., Bellucco, F. T., Christofolini, D. M., Mancini, T. I., Ribeiro-dos-Santos, Â. K., Santos, S. E., de Jesus Mari, J., Bressan, R. A., Melaragno M. I. & de Arruda Cardoso Smith, M. (2010) 'The UFD1L rs5992403 polymorphism is associated with age at onset of schizophrenia', *Journal of Psychiatric Research*, vol. 44, no. 15, pp. 1113–1115. doi:10.1016/j.jpsychires.2010.04.008.

Penttilä, J., Paillére-Martinot, M. -L., Martinot, J. -L., Mangin, J. -F., Burke, L., Corrigall, R., Frangou, S. & Cachia, A. (2008) 'Global and temporal cortical folding in patients with early-onset schizophrenia', *Journal of the American Academy of Child & Adolescent Psychiatry*, vol. 47, no. 10, pp. 1125–1132. doi:10.1097/CHI.0b013e3181825aa7.

Puig, O., Penadés, R., Baeza, I., Sánchez-Gistau, V., De la Serna, E., Fonrodona, L., Andrés-Perpiñá, S., Bernardo, M. & Castro-Fornieles, J. (2012) 'Processing speed and executive functions predict real-world everyday living skills in adolescents with early-onset schizophrenia', *European Child & Adolescent Psychiatry*, vol. 21, no. 6, pp. 315–326. doi:10.1007/s00787-012-0262-0.

Reichert, A., Kreiker, S., Mehler-Wex, C. & Warnke, A. (2008) 'The psychopathological and psychosocial outcome of early-onset schizophrenia: preliminary data of a 13-year follow-up', *Child And Adolescent Psychiatry And Mental Health*, vol. 2, no. 6. doi:10. 1186/1753-2000-2-6.

Remschmidt, H. & Theisen, F. (2012) 'Early-onset schizophrenia', *Neuropsychobiology*, vol. 66, no. 1, pp. 63–69. doi:10.1159/000338548.

Rhinewine, J. P., Lencz, T., Thaden, E. P., Cervellione, K. L., Burdick, K. E., Henderson, I., Bhaskar, S., Keehlisen, L., Kane, J., Kohn, N., Fisch, G. S., Bilder, R. M. & Kumra, S. (2005) 'Neurocognitive profile in adolescents with early-onset schizophrenia: clinical correlates', *Biological Psychiatry*, vol. 58, no. 9, pp. 705–712. doi:10.1016/j.biopsych.2005.04.031.

Robb, A. S., Carson, W. H., Nyilas, M., Ali, M., Forbes, R. A., Iwamoto, T., Assunção-Talbott, S., Whitehead, R. & Pikalov, A. (2010) 'Changes in Positive and Negative Syndrome Scale—derived hostility factor in adolescents with schizophrenia treated with aripiprazole: post hoc analysis of randomized clinical trial data', *Journal of Child and Adolescent Psychopharmacology*, vol. 20, no. 1, pp. 33–38. doi:10.1089/cap.2008.0163.

Romm, K. L., Rosenberg, J. I., Berg, A. O., Barrett, E. A., Faerden, A., Argartz, I., Andreassen, O. A. & Melle, I. (2010) 'Depression and depressive symptoms in first episode psychosis', *Journal of Nervous and Mental Disease*, vol. 198, no. 1, pp. 67–71. doi:10.1097/NMD.0b013e3181c81fc0.

Rowe, D. L., Robinson, P. A., Rennie, C. J., Harris, A. W., Felmingham, K. L., Lazzaro, I. L. & Gordon, E. (2004) 'Neurophysiologically-based mean-field modelling of tonic cortical activity in post-traumatic stress disorder (PTSD), schizophrenia, first episode schizophrenia and attention deficit hyperactivity disorder (ADHD)', *Journal of Integrative Neuroscience*, vol. 3, no. 4, pp. 453–487.

Russell, A. T., Bott, L. & Sammons, C. (1989) 'The phenomenology of schizophrenia occurring in childhood', *Journal of the American Academy of Child & Adolescent Psychiatry*, vol. 28, no. 3, pp. 399–407. doi:10.1097/00004583-198905000-00017.

Rutter, M. (1972) 'Childhood schizophrenia reconsidered', *Journal of Autism & Childhood Schizophrenia*, vol. 2, no. 4, pp. 315–337. doi:10.1007/bf01537622.

Schothorst, P. F., Emck, C. & van Engeland, H. (2006) 'Characteristics of early psychosis', *Comprehensive Psychiatry*, vol. 47, no. 6, pp. 438–442. doi:10.1016/j.comppsych. 2006.03.003.

Sikich, L. (2008) 'Efficacy of atypical antipsychotics in early-onset schizophrenia and other psychotic disorders', *The Journal of Clinical Psychiatry*, vol. 69, no. (Suppl 4), pp. 21–25.

Sowell, E. R., Levitt, J., Thompson, P. M., Holmes, C. J., Blanton, R. E., Kornsand, D. S., Caplan, R., McCracken, J., Asarnow, R. & Toga, A. W. (2000) 'Brain abnormalities in early-onset schizophrenia spectrum disorder observed with statistical parametric mapping of structural magnetic resonance images', *The American Journal of Psychiatry*, vol. 157, no. 9, pp. 1475–1484. doi:10.1176/appi.ajp.157.9.1475.

Spencer, E. K., Kafantaris, V., Padron-Gayol, M. V. & Rosenberg, C. R. (1992) 'Haloperidol in schizophrenic children: Early findings from a study in progress', *Psychopharmacology Bulletin*, vol. 28, no. 2, pp. 183–186.

Spina, E., Avenoso, A., Scordo, M. G., Ancione, M., Madia, A., Gatti, G. & Perucca, E. (2002) 'Inhibition of Risperidone metabolism by fluoxetine in patients with schizophrenia: a Clinically Relevant pharmacokinetic drug interaction', *Journal of Clinical Psychopharmacology*, vol. 22, no. 4, pp. 419–423.

Stafford, R. L. (2006) 'Regulating off-label drug use — rethinking the role of the FDA', *The New England Journal of Medicine*, vol. 358, pp. 1427–1429.

Tang, J., Liao, Y., Zhou, B., Tan, C., Liu, T., Hao, W., Hu, D. & Chen, X. (2010) 'Abnormal anterior cingulum integrity in first episode, early-onset schizophrenia: A diffusion tensor imaging study', *Brain Research*, vol. 1343, pp. 199–205. doi:10.1016/j.brainres.2010.04.083.

The Medicated Child, Introduction. (2009). Retrieved from http://www.pbs.org/wgbh/pages/frontline/medicatedchild/etc/synopsis.html

Thomsen, P. H. (1996) 'Schizophrenia with childhood and adolescent onset—a nationwide register-based study', *Acta Psychiatrica Scandinavica*, vol. 94, no. 3, pp. 187–193.

U.S. Department of Education. (2003) *25th Report to Congress on the Implementation of the Individuals with Disabilities Education Act. Office of Special Education and Rehabilitative Services*. Retrieved from http://www2.ed.gov/about/reports/annual/osep/2003/25th-vol-1.pdf

U.S. Department of Education. (2008) *30th Report to Congress on the Implementation of the Individuals with Disabilities Education Act.* Office of Special Education and Rehabilitative Services. Retrieved from http://www2.ed.gov/about/reports/annual/osep/2008/parts-b-c/30th-idea-arc.pdf

Walder, D. J., Seidman, L. J., Cullen, N., Su, J., Tsuang, M. T. & Goldstein, J. M. (2006) 'Sex differences in language dysfunction in schizophrenia', *The American Journal of Psychiatry*, vol. 163, no. 3, pp. 470–477. doi:10.1176/appi.ajp.163.3.470.

Whitaker, R. (2004) 'The case against antipsychotic drugs: a 50-year record of doing more harm than good', *Medical Hypotheses*, vol. 62, no. 1, pp. 5–13.

Wozniak, J. R., Block, E. E., White, T., Jensen, J. B. & Schulz, S. C. (2008) 'Clinical and neurocognitive course in early-onset psychosis: A longitudinal study of adolescents with schizophrenia-spectrum disorders', *Early Intervention in Psychiatry*, vol. 2, no. 3, pp. 169–177.

Michelle Gibson

ANALYSIS OF SOCIAL WORK PRACTICE: FOUCAULT AND FEMALE BODY IMAGE IN THERAPY

The cultural discourse of the female body is riddled with language of management for the individual and the practitioner. Social work practice with body image concerns calls for a best practice of cognitive behavioural therapy (CBT). CBT's focus on the maladaptive cognitions of the individual ignores the larger structural forces that lead to the development of body image, and also the structural forces present in the therapy room. Using a Foucauldian lens, drawing from personal and professional experience, and current literature, this article seeks to criticize the dominant discourse of traditional practice for negative body image in social work. This article seeks to critique the individualistic, surveillance and self-management practices of CBT for women experiencing negative body image. A narrative and social justice oriented approach to practice in the arena of body image that includes a socio-cultural analysis of the issue, reflexivity of the practitioner and an appreciation of resistance is taken. Limitations are outlined in recognition of the organizational barriers reflexive workers may encounter and the often-daily tension between best practice and ethical practice within which social workers must practice.

Discourses demand and produce real effects on people, especially their bodies.

(Foote & Frank, 1999, p. 172)

Introduction

According to Amigot and Pujal (2009),

> the Foucauldian analysis of power pushes us to analyse the inherent tension between subjection and the agency that repeatedly produces corporeality and forms of the subject without determining them, but also without allowing an imaginary space of absolute freedom and exteriority to historical and social conditions of its emergence. (p. 652)

This quote is provided as forethought of the aim of this paper on the construction of the female body in therapy and the treatment of body image disorder by therapists. As a woman socialized in western culture, I can attest to the pressure placed upon women to fit within a narrow ideal of what it means to be beautiful. I describe this experience as the navigation of dominant discourse between how I ought to look based on cultural standards and the personal struggle to attain this standard. As I emerged into young womanhood, fashion magazines became a major focus of adolescent attention and I would envision how I could change my appearance to fit within these cultural images. As my body changed, I fought against this restricting food intake and comparing my body to others. Through the images bombarding my adolescent self, I felt immense pressure to fit into a rigid model of what a woman ought to be.

My scope of experience lies within work as a Social Worker who facilitates therapy with individual. Before discussing the issue of body image dissatisfaction, it is important to first deconstruct issues related to therapy. There are many avenues from which one can approach therapy; I approach therapy from a feminist and postmodern position that aims to challenge a therapeutic positioning that reinforce problems as individually oriented instead of approaching problems as socially created. The passion I feel about this experience has transitioned to experience in social work practice. In conversations with women in therapy, they have shared accounts of daily body dissatisfaction. Their stories elucidate elements of my own story, particularly the feeling that there is an immense force influencing women to attain a physical beauty that often seems unrealistic. Research on this topic evidences the statements of women sharing stories in therapy. Markula (2001) concluded, 'body dissatisfaction among women had become so prevalent that, according to some medical researchers, it can be considered a normal part of the female experience' (p. 170). I posit there are two sources of knowledge: socio-cultural and medical, that act to create ideas about gender and bodies. With such a growing presence of women with body dissatisfaction, medical discourse has prescribed symptomology to the concern. Symptoms of body image dissatisfaction include time-consuming and emotionally-upsetting thoughts, grooming and comparisons to others (Wilhelm *et al.*, 2010, p. 241). Greenberg and Wilhelm (2010) wrote of the many negative effects of body image including impacts on sexual functioning and quality of life (p. 237). Body image dissatisfaction is a prevalent issue affecting most women throughout their life experience as evidenced by personal and professional experience and research.

Foote and Frank (1999) title a section of their writing 'therapy after Foucault', this is an accurate description of what this paper hopes to present (p. 158). In conducting research on body image, most findings related to treatment of body image dissatisfaction from a psychological lens influenced by medical and socio-cultural discourse. This lens includes focusing on the individual as the locus for change and monitoring behaviours, both by the client and the therapist. Presently, I facilitate therapy women who experience body image dissatisfaction. The evidence-based practice suggested to approach this issue is cognitive behavioural therapy (CBT), which will be addressed later in greater detail. Inspired by learnings of Foucauldian theory and understanding one's relationship to their body as being shaped by psychological, social and cultural factors, I questioned the role of power in CBT with women affected by body image dissatisfaction. I pondered the possibility of moving beyond the focus from the individual, and asking what role resistance presents within an alternative approach. This paper aims to provide an analysis of the present psychological model of treatment of body image dissatisfaction from a Foucauldian perspective. To do this, first, an evaluation of the current practice model will be presented. This section hopes to address the beliefs that underlie the construction of the problem of body image dissatisfaction in therapy. This exploration will include the role of therapy as a technology of the self, and concepts of individualization, surveillance, and therapy as a form of governmentality as applied to therapeutic practice. Second, an outline of alternative approaches to therapy with women who experience body image dissatisfaction will be presented using Foucauldian theory. An introduction to other approaches to body image dissatisfaction that might be addressed in therapy will be explored. This presentation will encourage a focus on socio-cultural factors in therapy through the concept of docile bodies, the importance of reflection for practitioners and exploring the role of resistance in therapy. Finally, implications and larger questions will be addressed in relation to the role of therapy in working with women who experience dissatisfaction with their bodies and recommendations will be identified. This paper, proposes reflection on present social work practice to include Foucauldian concepts that encourage identification of power relations and a holistic practice approach. The alternative approach presented is not a replacement for the traditional model; rather, it should be viewed as a suggestion for greater reflective, honest and client-centred practice.

The discourse of the female body in therapy

Technologies of the self

I introduce the concept of technology of the self as a key component to the proposal of this section. Foucault (1988b) acknowledged that therapy is a transformation of the individual. He described technologies of the self as therapy which

> permit individuals to effect by their own means or with the help of others a certain number of operations on their own bodies and souls, thoughts, conduct, and way of being, so as to transform themselves in order to attain a certain state of happiness, purity, wisdom, perfection, or immortality. (p. 18)

Therapy is, therefore, a process of addressing perceived issues in order to gain a positive outcome. Therapy is a technology of the self, according to Foucault, and is a common practice in identifying and treating body image dissatisfaction. Technologies of the self can act to uphold the dominant discourse or it can encourage resistance. I propose the current framework of treatment does the former. Professionals who maintain dominant discourse mediate technologies of the self, and social workers fulfil this role.

Individualization

Foucault (1973) stated 'medicine places the problem of disease on the individual body, fixing their investigative gaze on the body's signs and symptoms to determine its pathological state' (as cited in Markula, 2001, p. 172). Therapy focusing on body image dissatisfaction typically employs techniques that emphasize the role of the individual. In the pathologization of body dissatisfaction, the focus is placed upon the individual's ability to manage symptoms; if symptoms are unmanageable, therapeutic intervention is required. CBT is recommended as the means of addressing body image dissatisfaction. CBT 'focus(es) on the factors that maintain the patient's preoccupation and distress with their body image' (Veale, 2010, p. 336). In practice experience with CBT, the beginning stage of treatment typically involves individualizing the CBT treatment model. This means mapping problem thought patterns relating to distress due to body image dissatisfaction. Potential questions involved in the process are outlined by Phillips (2010) and are focused solely on the individual. These questions include (in suggested sequence): Are you worried about your appearance in any way? What aspects of your appearance do you dislike? How much distress do these concerns cause you? Do your concerns interrupt other areas of your life? (p. 320). These questions do not include language that might suggest body image dissatisfaction is greater than an individual pathological issue. Rather the questions suggest it is an issue solely of the individual's inability to manage body dissatisfaction.

The successful treatment of body image dissatisfaction is the client addressing *their* thoughts and *their* feelings towards their body. Behavioural change would accompany successful CBT treatment. Through focusing only on the client's thought process and behaviour, I argue, CBT is a mechanism of individualization. This individualization places emphasis on the client as the means of change to 'correct the individual's attitude of her self' and therefore, 'relegates responsibility for behaviour to individual patients' (Markula, 2001, pp. 170–172). The purpose of this individualization in therapy is to prevent dissent from the present socio-cultural discourse of women's bodies. Simplicity is achieved in targeting the individual and enforcing the idea of an abnormal pathology, rather than addressing the wider socio-cultural forces involved in constructing the concern. In not questioning larger constructions of body image dissatisfaction in women, the client is the only problem which is arguably much more manageable to the practitioner and to society.

Surveillance

The panopticon is 'a mechanism of surveillance' in which one has full view of the other behaviours; thus, the other is always watched (Moffatt, 1999, p. 224). Panopticon refers, in therapy, to the surveillance of the client extending beyond the observations made in an appointment. According to Tretheway (1999), 'women's bodies are on display, available to the "gaze" of both male and female disciplinarians'. She continued to argue that it is no surprise that 'women engage in self-surveillance and work hard at disciplining and normalizing their own bodies and selves' (p. 446). Women outside of therapy engage in self-surveillance by attending to cultural messages that tell women to be 'normal' through dieting, grooming behaviours and internal pressures on their appearance. Therapy continues this surveillance, through encouragement of self-management of thoughts, feelings and behaviours. The aim of CBT is to address negative or distorted thought patterns and alter these to create a positive and effective behavioural change. CBT is structured to include self-monitoring of thoughts and behaviours by the client within and outside of therapy (Wilhelm *et al.*, 2010, p. 242).

Practice experience with self-monitoring with young women at a secondary school, included a diary in which the client was directed to write down the date, time, location, negative thoughts (about body and appearance) and the perceived cause of the thought. Another homework assignment is a food intake count for weight regulation and a daily weight monitor. The client struggling with misconceptions of size would record weight each day in order to have a valid measure of fluctuation. Homework assignments are meant to focus on individuals troubling thought patterns beyond the weekly, hour-long therapy session. Both of these assignments are an example of surveillance that goes beyond the therapeutic session to the intimate lives of clients.

Surveillance serves, not only, to place the emphasis of the problem on the individual, but also to ensure the client is always aware of the therapeutic gaze. The panopticon allows therapists to monitor clients even out of direct sight. In support of this position, Brown *et al.* (2008) argued traditional treatment is 'embedded in dominant self-management discourse that focuses on body weight management and food intake and acts to perpetuate women's existing problematic focus on weight and eating' (pp. 92–93). Surveillance places further emphasis on the responsibility of the individual by continuing to ignore the larger discourse that creates and maintains body image dissatisfaction in women. Brown *et al.* (2008) continued by stating these discourses serve 'to control the body' (p. 102). Surveillance ensures the individual maintains standards of behaviour when away from the therapeutic relationship. The social worker encourages self-surveillance which acts to further the therapeutic gaze to the private lives of clients.

Governmentality

Governmentality is the 'management of individuals made possible by discourses claiming truth' (Foote & Frank, 1999, p. 161). Medical discourse permeates therapy by placing standards of health upon women of all ages. I refer to governmentality as the presence of state health models and upholds standards of the female body. Jones and Chandler (2007) wrote of Foucault's (1980, p. 39) concept of the technology of biopolitics referring to the 'points in which power reaches into every grain of individuals, touches their bodies and inserts itself into ... their everyday lives' (p. 150). Surveillance and enforcement control the body through powerful messages that pathologizes the negative relationship women have with their bodies. Body image dissatisfaction is defined through medical discourse by the American Psychiatric Association (1994) as a somatoform disorder in the DSM-IV (as cited in Wilhelm *et al.*, 2010, p. 241). This medicalization of female body image dissatisfaction is present in therapy when conducting an assessment and seeking a psychiatric referral. Not only does this categorization create a focus on an individual pathology, it also promotes a structured relationship with the therapist focusing on recommended healthy alternatives. The National Heart Lung and Blood Institute (US, 1998) recommended mental health professionals have knowledge of present healthy eating and exercise recommendations and determine the client's body mass index (BMI) in order to keep track of changes during treatment (in Sarwer, 2010, p. 279). Knowledge is also provided by the state through messages of what is healthy, and what is healthy according to this discourse, as evidenced by calculating BMI and exercise levels, is a thin female body. CBT reinforces the cultural beauty ideal that is one of the causes of body image dissatisfaction. In practice, I have calculated BMI's with clients and provided education around healthy eating. In this role, I have acted to further the idea that there is a normal body that is attainable through certain measures. This power is hidden within the therapeutic profession. According to Keenan (2001), 'disciplinary power operating systematically within a society and not from above' (p. 212). The therapeutic relationship is an example of the invisible power and discipline.

> The concept of social work as a dialogic, or relational, practice means that social workers in their assessments, interviews, and interventions are producing understandings of illness and health. We are, in effect, producing experiences of illness – power is indeed productive. (Phillips, 2007, p. 208)

Social work, in the profession's dialogical and interpersonal construct, acts as the force that maintains dominant discourse while doing so behind good intentions providing a space of invisibility.

Social work is a profession many individuals choose for noble reasons, but placing blame on the individual, surveillance of clients and upholding dominant discourse through a hidden narrative of what is healthy, is far from noble. Clients seek therapy as a space of acceptance and transformation. Markula (2001) wrote of Foucault's concept of 'the confessional mode' which acts to promote the worker to an authority that assesses and diagnoses the client, thus passing judgement (p. 175). The authority of therapist has been outlined as passing judgement and being grounded in a place of power. Social work utilizes this power through a normalizing gaze, which acts to 'create a field of comparison as individual acts are compared to a whole and to one another in a hierarchical, value-laden construction that outlines an average, and defines the bounds of the external limits' (Keenan, 2001, p. 213). The average, the ideal construct, is enforced through technologies of the self to encourage surveillance, self-management, ideas of normality and discipline of the individual. I argue this enforcement is practiced to uphold the current discourse and also to produce norm-abiding women. These women strive to attain the construct put forth by discourse through self-control.

A Foucauldian alternative to practice

Advancing from current best practice approaches, the second section of this paper seeks to ask how else social workers might approach practice. Specifically, the hope is to address how Foucault's concepts and postmodern theory could provide an alternative practice for social workers providing therapy to women with body image dissatisfaction. Burr (1995) wrote 'to understand power inequities in society properly, we need to examine how discursive practices serve to create and uphold particular forms of social life' (p. 63). Within this section, an exploration of concepts of the Foucauldian idea of docile bodies, reflection by workers in practice and the role of resistance in therapy are covered. As aforementioned, these alternatives are explored as suggestions for improved practice not as a guide to replace current practice, and also to explore where therapy might develop in the future in work with women experiencing body image dissatisfaction.

Docile bodies

The first issue in social work practice focusing on body image is the individualization of body image dissatisfaction, which ignores the larger, socio-cultural context from which body image dissatisfaction may be analysed. The Foucauldian concept of 'docile bodies' is utilized to present the argument that women's bodies are made docile in therapy and in society through pathologizing practices (Tretheway, 1999, p. 424). As women are pathologized and controlled in therapy, their bodies are managed. Docile bodies reflect women who are under this control. The social and cultural forces on women are numerous and far from invisible. Bordo (as cited in Markula, 2001, p. 168) describes the successful modern consumer as the slender female body. This body is able to self-master slenderness while still able to consume food. Bordo (1989) called this the bodily discourse, and states that it is through this discourse we are taught rules which tell women what clothes, body shape, behaviours and expressions are required (p. 17). Women are socialized to attain a narrow measure of attractiveness to be successful; women's bodies are thus controlled by the dominant discourse. 'The more a girl assumes her status as feminine, the more she takes herself to be fragile and immobile, and the more she actively enacts her own body inhibition' (Young, 1990, p. 154). Women are made docile within western culture, and therapeutic practice that individualizes the issue furthers the discipline of the female body. Women who seek treatment, within the above-mentioned common practice, are treated as having a personal failure, unable to mediate the force of culture and the psyche, and therefore unable to control their body.

Markula (2001) asked provided questions about responsibility in culture that can be applied to therapy as well. She asked, 'How are we persuaded to look for individual solutions to an "illness" whose cause is allegedly social?' (p. 169). I posit that through moving away from the medicalized view of body image dissatisfaction as a disorder to viewing body image dissatisfaction as a process of internalization shaped from social and cultural factors, the responsibility moves away from the client to a holistic view of the issue. Women with body image dissatisfaction can move beyond the control of dominant discourse with an alternative therapeutic lens. 'A narrative approach helps women begin to understand how discourses in the wider social context support the problem description they have of themselves and aims to help externalize the problem from the person' (Brown *et al.*, 2008, p. 97). Through externalizing the problem, narrative therapists allow the client to move from having a disorder to living in a disordered culture. This is not only freeing, and empowering to the client, but allows the therapist to move away from the therapeutic focus that places blame on the individual. Externalizing conversations (White & Epston, 1990; White, 2007; Duvall & Beres, 2011) stop the person from being disabled by the problem and disrupt pathologizing language. Language is used that does not attribute body image to the individual, for example: Tell me more about how negative body image affects you? When does negative body image present itself? To further this, I often have clients name the problem. For example, a young woman described her negative body image, or body image disorder (BID), as a broken mirror. She said when she looks in the different mirror she sees a different person, a person she does not like. Naming the problem allowed me to speak to the individual without applying the BID to her directly. The broken mirror became a word synonymous with body image.

Reflection

Reflection on the part of the therapist working with women affected by body image dissatisfaction is the recognition of the power involved in social work. This power is not hierarchical; power is present in all of the interactions and relations of the therapist to the client. Burr (1995) wrote of Foucault's notions of power, and states 'power resides everywhere' (p. 70). Although social workers may attempt to limit the power present in interactions with clients, practices such as CBT for body image dissatisfaction remind us that power can be found in therapy. Barns (2003) concluded social workers have often 'sought to regulate and mediate women's interactions with the social, economic, and political world' (p. 149). When the worker encourages the client to take responsibility for their feelings of dissatisfaction with their body and enforce medical and socio-cultural models for health, the worker is utilizing power to maintain dominant discourse. The change needed comes in the form of reflection in practice, direct reflection on the force of power in the therapeutic relationship. For 'experienced therapists periodic analysis of how dominant trends are influencing perceptions of normality' (Keenan, 2001, p. 255). Workers could become empowered to analyse the many levels of truth in therapeutic practice. Therapy is no longer the knowing helping the disordered; it must become a mechanism of reflection in order to truly honour the fundamental values of social work. How can practice speak to the unique stories present in the experience body mage dissatisfaction? How can practitioners begin to move away from a standardized model and to a model based on the client's experience? There is power in therapy, but it need not dominate interactions with the client. Irving (1999) writes an account of the fluidity of social work. He states:

> Saying words, as long as there are any, and speaking the multitudinous truths of life however troubling until they find us, until they recreate us, may enable social work to withstand the sharp gusts that shake our souls at modernity's end. (p. 48)

The importance of reflection in social work practice focused on body image dissatisfaction is twofold. First, reflection creates an arena for growth in the profession of social work that allows a shift from dominant discourse to ways of knowing based on multiple truths. This is a shift away from governmentality, of individualizing and surveillance. The reflective worker is one that examines the reality of the client from various standpoints. Second, and what will be analysed in more detail in the following paragraph, is the effect alternative practices will have on the client. 'As alternative narratives emerge, clients can separate themselves from their unhelpful dominant stories and experience agency and a capacity' (Brown *et al.*, 2008, p. 96). The client, provided a space with alternative narratives, is provided power to question why a certain body ideal is necessary. 'If we can understand the origins of our current ways of understanding ourselves, we can begin to question their legitimacy and resist them' (Burr, 1995, p. 69). I argue, reflection and resistance on the part of the practitioner, leads to reflection and resistance in the client.

Resistance

'Foucault insists that the body as constructed is not incapable of resisting or defying some of the demands of that discourse' (Cahill, 2000, p. 47). In the first section of this paper, I proposed that social work maintains discourse through mechanisms that encourage control and surveillance in clients. I posit that resistance can always be found in power relations and question how therapy can encourage this resistance. As women are made docile and are controlled by the construction of the female body in the dominant discourse, a power to counter this is present. Foucault believed that 'just as power is directed first and foremost toward the body, so resistance begins in the body' (Foote & Frank, 1999, p. 175). To adopt a stance of resistance, the view of body image dissatisfaction rooted in knowledge from dominant medical and socio-cultural discourses must be challenged. The psychological discourse promoting CBT identifies control over behaviour as evidenced by the homework assignments assessing food intake, weight, and negative thoughts. Behaviour, as viewed through a psychological gaze, is an expression of abnormal thoughts that are to be altered with therapy. Could this behaviour be viewed as a means of using the body for the purpose of self-control that is resisting food, focusing on the negative or eating too much? Could this be the client resisting the dominant narrative that tells women to control their food intake, restrict their size, adopt an ideal of beauty and to not complain? Gremillion (2003) found that the medical discourse 'fails to acknowledge and undermine the way women resource their bodies to maintain a sense of autonomy and self control' (in Brown *et al.*, 2008, p. 94). An alternative to the these discourses lies within reflection of how these behaviours are analysed in therapy and question the role of resistance and resilience of women to counter the discourse that is seeking control over the body.

As mediators of social justice, social workers are the directors of this resistance and practitioners play another role in resistance within therapy. While the practice of CBT focuses on control of thoughts and behaviour through therapy, there is an opportunity to view therapy as a space for alternative thought. Therapy can then provide a space for exploration of the causes of body image dissatisfaction, the implications of dominant discourse on the female body and the effects of the impositions of these standards. Feminist practice espouses such values by encouraging 'empowerment, social change, and self direction' (Brown *et al.*, 2008, p. 95). Advocating for self-direction and social change is encouraging resistance from the discourses that seeks to create and maintain docile women. In conversations with women, I have often posed questions that shift from the standardized format of CBT, to an analysis and deconstruction of control and management. Resistance in practice does not appear as a rebellion but rather as questioning. Magazines, television shows and movies are readily available as basis for beginning to question the standard construction of beauty and how this relates to body image dissatisfaction in women. Creating a picture of what an ideal woman looks like and deconstructing how and why this is idea is present is an example of this practice. This cultural analysis of body image dissatisfaction promotes exploration beyond the self to the social and cultural elements of the issue. Many young women tell stories of beauty as a concrete standard, beauty as unattainable yet desired. Through the deconstruction of photos and images, the therapist and the client 'disrupt the idea that there is one objective truth universal to all people and reveals the "political" or non-neutral nature of the ideas' (Brown *et al.*, 2008, p. 96). Foucault (1988a, 1988b) wrote that control over bodies is never complete, invariably resistance is present or there would be no relations of power. It is important for social workers to facilitate conversations that critique dominant discourse within therapy, while also facilitating conversations that encourage resistance outside of therapy. Some questions I use to encourage bringing forward developments in therapy are: What has shifted in your view of your self and the world based on our conversation today? Based on this, what might these shifts make possible for you? Are there people in your life who you would like to share these shifts with? Practitioners must, therefore, be cognizant to the presence of resistance and invaluable, importance of resistance as a means of empowerment.

Limitations and further questioning

The belief in multiple truths is encouraged as an alternative practice and this belief should also be applied to support the validity of CBT practice in working with women experiencing body image dissatisfaction. After outlining issues of current CBT practice with women experiencing body image dissatisfaction and also describing alternatives for practice, there are unanswered questions and no 'right' way to practice. The analysis of CBT through a Foucauldian lens and the suggestions for alternative practice are key in raising questions about the role of social work through a postmodernist lens. What was not addressed in this paper is whether the role of social work is suited to practice in support of discourse. Does it adhere to social work values to engage in such hierarchal power relations with clients? On the other hand, one might question the legitimacy of a social worker who imposes postmodernist ideas upon a client when there are evidence-based practices that could be drawn upon. In raising questions of resistance, control, surveillance, etc., is this another expression of power? In the conclusion of this paper, I provide a Foucauldian dismantling of CBT and offer some thoughts for post modernist practice. These thoughts are not mentioned to replace the effectiveness of the present practice. I do not suggest there is an alternative model that could act as a complete therapeutic manual, but I also do not rule out the possibility of an alternative therapeutic model. Given the time and space constraints of this paper, such a model could not be provided or explored. Instead, I hope questions have been raised in regards to faults of the current practice and that a space has been created for consideration of alternative practice. In future research, a focus on social work practice from a Foucauldian and postmodern lens are important in giving voice to alternative spaces for therapy. In much day-to-day therapy, social workers may forget there is practice beyond manualized therapy, that questioning traditional approaches allow for critical analysis to occur. Where there is critical, analysis there is growth in skills and knowledge which lends to better practice with clients.

Conclusion

The aim of this paper is a proposal to practitioners to reflect on current therapeutic practice in approaching body image dissatisfaction with women. Foucault's concepts of technologies of the self, individuality, governmentality, surveillance, docile bodies, power and resistance have been described and addressed as they apply to present therapy and recommendations for future practice. Within social work practice, the worker is provided a power, through credentials and trust, to pass judgement and encourage adherence to structural and cultural norms. Therapeutic power permeates practice when practice focuses solely on the individual for cause of the presenting problem and the mechanism for change of the problem. Power is also present when practitioners encourage dominant ideals of healthy and beauty. Surveillance is conducive to the ideal in managing the client in therapy and also having the client self-manage outside of therapy. These Foucauldian concepts are explored to display the presence of power in therapy and raise questions of beneficiaries in this process. In focusing on the individual, it is certainly not the client who is receiving best treatment. The second section provides an exploration of alternatives to practice that focus on cultural and social elements of body image dissatisfaction and focus on faults in the worker not the client. Reflection of the worker is encouraged in order to remain critical in practice. An exploration of resistance in therapy and with body image issues in women presents a different view of the problem. Instead of the client being defined as difficult or disordered, a resistance perspective would view the client as gaining power in questioning appearance. The alternatives presented are to be viewed as a reinforcement for greater reflective, honest and client-centred practice. The goal is that the reader is left with questions and reflections on the current practice, and that hope is instilled for what practice could be in the future. In social work practice, I have often struggled for a balance between what is best practice (CBT) and what is value based practice in working with women who are affected by body image dissatisfaction. This is an area I am most passionate about because of personal and professional experience, and I struggle to refrain from concluding this paper with a definitive answer as to how practitioners should approach clients presenting with body image dissatisfaction. It is in this tension, between limits of the present practice and opportunities for future practice, that I believe the most useful, reflective thought emerges, and from this the most client-centred practice is developed. To conclude, I encourage practitioners to explore this tension when filling out an assessment form for a woman with body image dissatisfaction. I encourage workers to question why they are directly or indirectly encouraging bodies through their lines of questions and focus on therapy and encourage self-reflection about where our, as social workers, source of knowledge comes from and whose voices are represented within it. As it is when, as practitioners, we cease to question that their practice is uncritical, then they practice oppressively. When we practice in tension, in complicated spaces within which discourse is open to questioning, we are practicing critically and anti-oppressively.

References

American Psychiatric Association (1994) *Diagnostic and Statistical Manual of Mental Disorders*, 4th ed., Author, Washington, DC.

Amigot, P. & Pujal, M. (2009) 'On power, freedom, and gender: a fruitful tension between Foucault and feminism', *Theory & Psychology*, vol. 19, no. 5, pp. 646–669.

Barns, A. (2003) 'Social work, young women, and femininity', *Affilia*, vol. 18, no. 2, pp. 148–164.

Bordo, S. (1989) 'The body and the reproduction of femininity', in *Gender, Body, Knowledge*, eds A. Jaggar & S. Bordo, Rutgers University Press, New Brunswick, NJ, pp. 13–33.

Brown, C. G., Weber, S. & Ali, S. (2008) 'Women's body talk: a feminist narrative approach', *Journal of Systemic Therapies*, vol. 27, no. 2, pp. 92–104.

Burr, V. (1995) *An Introduction to Social Constructionism*, Routledge, New York, NY.

Cahill, A. J. (2000) 'Foucault, rape, and the construction of the feminine body', *Hypatia*, vol. 15, no. 1, pp. 43–63.

Duvall, J. & Beres, L. (2011) *Innovations in Narrative Therapy: Connecting Practice, Training, and Research*, WW Norton & Company, New York, NY.

Foote, C. & Frank, A. W. (1999) 'Foucault and therapy: the disciplining of grief', in *Reading Foucault for Social Work*, eds A. Chambon, A. Irving & L. Epstein, Columbia University Press, New York, NY.

Foucault, M. (1973) *The Birth of the Clinic: An Archeology of Medical Perception*, Pantheon, New York, NY.

Foucault, M. (1980) 'Prison talk: interview by J.J. Brochier', in *Power/Knowledge: Selected Interviews and Other Writings, 1972–77*, ed. C. Gordon, Pantheon Books, New York, NY, pp. 37–54.

Foucault, M. (1988a) 'On power', in *Politics, Philosophy, Culture: Interviews and Other Writings, 1977–84*, ed. L. D. Kritzman, Routledge, New York, NY.

Foucault, M. (1988b) 'Technologies of the self', in *Technologies of the Self: A Seminar with Michel Foucault*, eds L. H. Martin, H. Gutman & P. H. Hutton, University of Massachusetts Press, Amherst, MA, pp. 16–49.

Greenberg, J. L. & Wilhelm, S. (2010) 'Special series: cognitive behavioral treatment of body image disorder', *Cognitive and Behavioral Practice*, vol. 17, pp. 237–240.

Gremillion, H. (2003) *Feeding Anorexia: Gender and Power at a Treatment Center*, Duke University Press, Durham, NC.

Irving, A. (1999) 'Waiting for Foucault: social work and the multitudinous truth(s) of life', in *Reading Foucault for Social Work*, eds A. Chambon, A. Irving & L. Epstein, Columbia University Press, New York, NY, pp. 27–50.

Jones, J. B. & Chandler, S. (2007) 'Surveillance and regulation control of women casino workers' bodies', *Affilia: Journal of Women and Social Work*, vol. 22, no. 2, pp. 150–162.

Keenan, E. K. (2001) 'Using Foucault's "disciplinary power" and "resistance: in cross-cultural psychotherapy"', *Clinical Social Work Journal*, vol. 29, no. 3, pp. 211–227.

Markula, P. (2001) 'Beyond the perfect body: women's body image distortion in fitness magazines', *Journal of Sport and Social Issues*, vol. 25, no. 2, pp. 158–179.

Moffatt, K. (1999) 'Surveillance and government of the welfare recipient', in *Reading Foucault for Social Work*, eds A. Chambon, A. Irving & L. Epstein, Columbia University Press, New York, NY, pp. 219–245.

National Heart, Blood, and Lung Institute (1998) *Clinical Guidelines on the identification, Evaluation, and Treatment of Overweight and Obesity in the United States: The Evidence Report*, No. 98-4083, National Institutes of Health, Washington, DC.

Phillips, C. (2007) 'Pain(ful) subjects: regulated bodies in medicine and social work', *Qualitative Social Work*, vol. 6, no. 2, pp. 197–212.

Phillips, K. A. (2010) 'Assessment and differential diagnosis for Body Dysmorphic Disorder', *Psychiatric Annals*, vol. 40, no. 7, pp. 317–324.

Sarwer, D. B. (2010) 'Invited commentary special series: cognitive behavioral therapy for Body Image Disorders', *Cognitive and Behavioral Practice*, vol. 17, pp. 278–282.

Tretheway, A. (1999) 'Disciplined bodies: women's embodied identities at work', *Organization Studies*, vol. 20, no. 3, pp. 423–450.

Veale, D. (2010) 'Cognitive behavioral therapy for Body Dysmorphic Disorder', *Psychiatric Annals*, vol. 40, no. 7, pp. 333–340.

White, M. (2007) *Maps of Narrative Practice*, Norton, New York, NY.

White, M. & Epston, D. (1990) *Narrative Means to Therapeutic Ends*, Norton, New York, NY.

Wilhelm, S., Buhlmann, U., Hayward, L. C., Greenberg, J. L. & Dimaite, R. (2010) 'A cognitive behavioral treatment approach for Body Dysmorphic Disorder', *Cognitive and Behavioral Practice*, vol. 17, pp. 241–247.

Young, I. M. (1990) *Throwing Like a Girl and Other Essays in Feminist Philosophy and Social Theory*, Indiana University Press, Bloomington, IN.

Maria Liegghio and Prableen Jaswal

POLICE ENCOUNTERS IN CHILD AND YOUTH MENTAL HEALTH: COULD STIGMA INFORMED CRISIS INTERVENTION TRAINING (CIT) FOR PARENTS HELP?

Recently in Canada the issue of police encounters among persons living with a mental health issue has received considerable public attention; however, the focus has been primarily on the experiences of adults and not of children and youth. In this paper, we explore police encounters in child and youth mental health by presenting the outcomes of 14 qualitative interviews conducted with seven caregivers and seven siblings and two focus groups conducted with eight caregivers about their experiences of having a child/sibling, 13–21 years old, living with a mental health issue. There were two main themes identified: (1) the need for police support to deescalate a high conflict situation involving a distressed child/sibling, and (2) the stigmatisation and criminalisation of the distressed child, parents and families. Based on these outcomes, a model of support is proposed whereby parents would be provided with crisis intervention training informed by an understanding of the stigma of mental illness as a structural condition of their personal experiences. Such training could provide caregivers with support for identifying and responding to crisis and for developing safety plans that may or may not involve police, but could minimise and/or divert the need for their involvement.

Introduction

Over recent years in Canada the issue of policing and police encounters among persons living with a mental health issue has received considerable public attention with numerous government inquests examining the deaths of adults living with a mental illness by police (Braidwood Commission, 2009; Eden, 2014; Iacobucci, 2014), as well as several national research initiatives aimed at improving the mental health and justice systems (Cotton & Coleman, 2008; Coleman & Cotton, 2010; Brink *et al.*, 2011; Chammartin *et al.*, 2011). Despite this increased attention, the focus of empirical research has been on the experiences of adults living with a mental health issue and not of children and youth. This lack of attention represents a significant gap in our academic and practice knowledge; thus, the aim of this paper is to examine the issue of policing and police encounters in child and youth mental health. In particular, we present the outcomes of 14 qualitative semi-structured interviews conducted independently with caregivers/parents[1] and siblings and two focus groups conducted with caregivers about their experiences of having a child/sibling between 13 and 21 years old living with a mental health issue.

An unexpected outcome to have emerged was the extent to which the families had involvement with police as a mental health intervention. In particular, there are two main themes: (1) the need for police support to deescalate a high conflict verbal and/or physical situation involving a distressed child, and (2) the stigmatisation and criminalisation of the distressed child, parents and families related to the police involvement. Based on these outcomes, a model of support is proposed whereby parents would be provided with crisis intervention training (CIT) informed by an understanding of the stigma of mental illness. We propose that such training could provide caregivers with important support for identifying and responding to crisis and for developing safety plans that may or may not involve police, but that could minimise and/or divert the need for their involvement.

Literature review

Police encounters in child and youth mental health

Generally, scholarship on policing and police encounters in child and youth mental health is very limited. Conservative estimates suggest that 15% (Kirby & Keon, 2006) or one in five (Shanley et al., 2008) Canadian children and youth live with a mental health issue. Currently in both policy and practice, there are limited (if any) reliable public statistics documenting the rate to which young people, and their caregivers and family members, encounter or use police services as an emergency mental health response. Moreover, the nature and reasons for police involvement (except for youth already involved in the justice system) are relatively unknown – representing a major limitation in our academic and professional knowledge. Largely the focus is of the experiences of adults for which estimates suggest that approximately 7–15% of police calls involve a person living with a mental illness (Cotton & Coleman, 2008) and that approximately 65% of adults newly admitted to inpatient and community psychiatric services had some sort of encounter with police (Brink et al., 2011). The reasons for police involvement included being a victim of crime, a suspect of crime, attempted suicide or for escorts to the hospital for psychiatric care (Cotton & Coleman, 2008; Coleman & Cotton, 2010).

Other studies included: exploring the perceptions adults with a mental health issue have of police and police interactions; detailing the education and training police officers, as first responders, receive about mental illness; and examining the human rights legislation affecting persons living with a mental health issue (Cotton & Coleman, 2008; Coleman & Cotton, 2010; Brink et al., 2011; Chammartin et al., 2011). More broadly, others have reported on the in/appropriateness of police approaches for intervening with psychiatrically distressed individuals (Morabito *et al.*, 2012), as well as the effectiveness of CIT for police on diverting adults away from the criminal justice system (Canada *et al.*, 2012; Coleman & Cotton, 2014). Based on adults' experiences, there are several important concerns discussed about policing and police encounters. These include the inappropriate use of force and physical restraints and the criminalisation of mental illness and of persons living with a mental illness (Fry *et al.*, 2002; Corrigan *et al.*, 2005; Watson *et al.*, 2008; Morabito *et al.*, 2012). The criminalisation of mental illness is cited as a major form of structural discrimination in which adults living with mental health issues are inappropriately treated by the criminal justice system instead of the mental health system (Corrigan *et al.*, 2005; Gur, 2010; Chaimowitz, 2012). As an issue the stigma of mental illness, in its various forms, is cited as a major barrier to accessing mental health services, as well as a serious factor that can negatively impact personal well-being and family relationships and functioning (Tuchman, 1996; Richardson, 2001; Hinshaw, 2005; Zimmerman, 2005; Samargia *et al.*, 2006; Moskos *et al.*, 2007; Koro-Ljungberg & Bussing, 2009; Munson *et al.*, 2009; O'Reilly *et al.*, 2009; Liegghio, 2013).[2]

As important as these contributions are, little attention is paid to police encounters occurring with children and youth living with a mental health issue. Instead, the experiences of young people are embedded or implied within other areas; for example, in research examining the referral to police and arrest rates among youth receiving mental health care (Vander Koep *et al.*, 1997; Robst *et al.*, 2013), and the mental health and/or substance use needs of already criminally involved or convicted youth (Carswell *et al.*, 2004; Erickson & Butters, 2005; Odgers *et al.*, 2005; Chassin, 2008; Townsend *et al.*, 2010). In a rather dated study, youth using community-based mental health services were nearly three times more likely to be referred to police, and generally, were more likely to be subsequently convicted for minor infractions, i.e. vandalism, trespassing and minor assaults/thefts (Vander Koep *et al.*, 1997). More recently, Robst *et al.* (2013) compared the arrest rates between young people receiving in-patient psychiatric, group home and foster home mental health treatment, and found youth in group home settings had higher arrest rates than those in in-patient psychiatric settings. Among the reasons suggested for the differences were the policies and practices in different settings with staff within group homes being more likely to involve police. In addition, Robst *et al.* suggest that the higher rates may relate to responding police officers over time becoming de-sensitised to the mental health issues of the young person, and thus may be more likely to lay charges on subsequent interactions.

In research examining the mental health needs of criminally convicted youth Odgers *et al.* (2005) report an estimate 20% of young people (two-thirds of males and three-quarters of females) met the criteria for at least one diagnosis of a 'mental illness'. The rates shift higher when examining type of disorder (e.g. approximately 30% of youth met the criteria for depression; 30% for anxiety; 90% for post-traumatic stress disorder and 50% for substance abuse issues). Although these findings were not directly about the experiences youth have of police encounters, they do imply the potential criminalisation and entrenchment of youth living with a mental health issue into the criminal justice system – a system ill-equipped to offer more than basic mental health care (Moskos *et al.*, 2007; Doulas & Lurigio, 2010).

To begin to establish the extent to which children and youth experiencing emotional, mental and psychological difficulties have encounters with police, Liegghio *et al.* (in press) conducted a secondary data analysis of intake statistics for an urban-based community child and youth mental health agency. The analysis found over a five-year period, from 2009 to 2014 there were 8920 intakes completed of children and youth from birth to 24 years old accessing mental health services. Of those children and youth, 1449 had police involvement at the time of intake. In other words, 16% or one in six children or youth accessing mental health services had police involvement. Towards understanding the reasons and nature of the involvement, the research reported here provides a qualitative description of the experiences young people living with a mental health issue have of police encounters from the perspectives of their caregivers and siblings.

Methodology

The research reported here was part of a larger study (refer to Liegghio, 2013) that used both qualitative and quantitative methods to explore self and family stigma in child and youth mental health from the perspectives of young people diagnosed with a mental health issue, caregivers and siblings. In this paper, we present the outcomes of the 14 qualitative, semi-structured interviews conducted independently with seven ($n = 7$) caregivers and seven ($n = 7$) siblings and two focus groups conducted with eight ($n = 8$) caregivers. There were a total of 22 participants. All the interviews and focus groups were guided by three questions focused on: (1) the ways caregivers and siblings perceived, interpreted and experienced their child's/sibling's mental health issue; (2) how those experiences shaped their sense of self as parents/siblings and on their sense of family; and (3) whether the experiences indicated stigma. Although the focus was not directly on encounters within the criminal justice system, the extent to which children and youth, caregivers and siblings had involvement with police was an unexpected outcome.

Purposive sampling was used to identify a non-random selection of caregivers and siblings. The criterion for inclusion was: caregivers with a child between 12 and 22 years old identified as having a mental health issue and siblings, 13–21 years old, living with or having lived within the previous two years with a brother or sister identified as having a mental health issue. The families had to be nearing the end of their mental health treatment. Siblings and caregivers experiencing an acute mental health crisis were excluded because, presumably, they were facing immediate circumstances that would make it difficult for them to participate and might have required more support than was possible within a research context.

Recruitment occurred through a community-based children's mental health service agency located in a large urban centre near Toronto, Canada. A letter of introduction was provided to frontline mental health workers to pass along to caregivers with children/siblings meeting the criterion for participation. The letter directed interested persons to contact the principal researcher (Maria) directly. Once contacted, caregivers and siblings with their caregivers were provided with the full details of the study: the purpose, the procedures, and the risks and benefits of participation. Siblings under 18 years old required the consent of their legal guardians to participate. Appropriate caregivers and siblings were invited to participate in interviews and/or focus groups. All the interviews and focus groups were conducted between January and August 2011. The interviews were each approximately one to one and half hours, and the focus groups were approximately one and half to two hours – each were audio taped and transcribed verbatim. Siblings and caregivers were provided with a $15.00 travel allowance and a $30.00 honorarium for recognition and appreciation of their time. Ethical approval was obtained through the Research Ethics Board at Wilfrid Laurier University, as well as the agency partner.

The data for analysis consisted of the demographic information collected about the participants and the transcripts of 14 interviews and 2 focus groups (16, $n = 16$ transcripts in total). Data analysis of the transcripts was an inductive process consisting of a thematic content analysis and based on the principles of grounded theory (Creswell, 1998; Strauss & Corbin, 1998). To ensure the rigour and trustworthiness of the findings, feedback on the initial concepts was obtained from at least one sibling and one caregiver through a verification process. In addition, to validate the category system an independent reviewer analysed segments of both a caregiver and sibling interview transcript (Burnard, 1991) using the same procedures. When presenting the findings, pseudonyms are used and identifying information is altered to protect the confidentiality of the caregivers, siblings and their family members. The following tables summarise the demographic information about the caregivers and siblings (see Tables 1 and 2).

Of the 15 caregivers, 2 had a child with one mental health diagnosis, 6 with two diagnoses and 7 with three or more diagnoses. Thirteen caregivers had a child actively using mental health services at the time of the interview and/or focus group with eight caregivers having a child with experiences of residential care or psychiatric hospitalisation. Of the seven siblings, one had a brother/sister with one mental health diagnosis, three with a brother/sister with two diagnoses and three with a brother/sister with three or more diagnoses. All seven siblings had a brother or sister that were actively using mental health services at the time of the interview, with four siblings having a brother or sister with experiences of residential care or psychiatric hospitalisation. The most prevalent mental health conditions the children/siblings were diagnosed to have included: attention deficit/hyperactivity disorder; anxiety, generalised anxiety or social anxiety; depression; bi-polar affective disorder; oppositional defiant disorder; and at least one episode of paranoia, delusions, psychosis or explosive aggression. The prevalence of these disorders was not surprising and was consistent with rates reported broadly in the literature for children and youth (Offord et al., 1998; Silk et al., 2000; Boyle & Willms, 2002; Shanley et al., 2008). In the next section, we present the outcomes to have emerged from the interviews and focus groups.

Outcomes

Police encounters from the perspectives of caregivers and siblings

Of the 22 caregivers and young siblings involved in the study, 60% ($n = 13$) had experiences of police involvement related to their child's/sibling's mental health issue (eight of the fifteen caregivers and five of the seven siblings)[3]. Although generalisations cannot be made due to the small sample size, this rate was consistent with those reported for adults (65%) (refer to Brink et al., 2011). There are two main themes identified: (1) the need for police support to deescalate a high conflict verbal and/or

TABLE 1 Caregiver demographic information

Total number of caregiver/participants	15	
Gender the caregiver/participants	2 = Male/fathers	13 = Female/mothers
Age range of caregiver/participants	44–55 years old (average age = 49)	
Citizenship	9 = Canadian born	
	6 = Born outside of Canada (migrated from South East Asia, Middle East, Caribbean, Africa, the USA. The number of years living in Canada ranged from 21 to 52 years)	
Race	10 = Caucasian	
	5 = Racialised (Black, Filipino, Middle East)	
Sexual orientation	13 = Heterosexual	
	2 = Lesbian, self-identified	
Highest grade completed	1 = Grade 9	
	4 = College or some college	
	10 = University or some university	
Annual family income	3 = Under $30,000	
	2 = $41,000 to $50,000	
	3 = $61,000 to $80,000	
	7 = over $80,000	
Relationship status of the caregivers	8 = Married/heterosexual	
	2 = Married/same-sex	
	2 = Separated/heterosexual	
	3 = Divorced/heterosexual	
Family composition	9 = Two parent family	
	6 = Single parent, female-headed, family	
Ages of identified child at the time of the focus group/interview	1 = 12 years old	
	1 = 13 years old	
	5 = 15 years old	
	3 = 16 years old	
	2 = 18 years old	
	2 = 19 years old	
	1 = 20 years old	

physical situation involving a distressed child/sibling, and (2) the stigmatisation and criminalisation of the child, parents and families.

Theme one: deescalate a high conflict situation involving a distressed child/sibling

Generally, family members call police services for support to intervene in mental health matters in order to: deescalate high conflict situations in which the young person is harming or threatening to harm themselves or others; because the young

TABLE 2 Sibling demographic information

Total number of sibling/participants	7	
Gender the sibling/participants	3 = Male	4 = Female
Ages of sibling/participants	13, 13, 14, 15, 16, 16, 21 years old	
	(average: 15 years old)	
Citizenship	7 = Canadian born	
Race	6 = Caucasian	
	1 = Black (African decent)	
Highest grade completed	2 = Grade 7	
	1 = Grade 8	
	1 = Grade 9	
	2 = Grade 10	
	1 = One year undergraduate university	
Annual family income as reported by	3 = Under $30,000	
caregivers	1 = $41,000 to $50,000	
	3 = Over $80,000	
Family composition	2 = Two parent family	
	5 = Single parent, female-headed family	
Gender of the brother/sister diagnosed with a mental health issue	6 = Brothers	1 = Sister
Ages of the brother/sister with the mental health issue at the time of the interview	12, 13, 15, 16, 16, 18, 22 years old	

person is accused of committing an illegal act; and, if required, to implement physical interventions, such as a physical restraint or an escort to the hospital for an emergency psychiatric assessment. Mothers, Ashley, Jeanette and Christine, as well as 16-year old sibling, Lindsay, describe the situations for which police were called for support.

> ASHLEY [mother]: This is scary because his mood, his mood has changed so much. One time he's very good, one time he's not. And that, as a parent, you are scared because sometimes you don't know what is going to happen, whether he's going to really get mad, it's like screaming, yelling, and it's scary.
>
> JEANETTE [mother]: The one day it was really scary, I mean he's [son] done things, I mean, with knives to himself or like holding her [sister's] hair, pulling it so hard. Like you know, and that's very scary, right. Like, or having to yell at her [sister] to go lock yourself in the bathroom ... He's threatened me with a knife before ... he had the knife to his throat, he said he was so mad at me for something, he's saying, 'oh, I am going to kill myself'.
>
> CHRISTINE [mother]: I've actually had to call the police ... he [son] was playing Xbox live [online video game] and his sister got on the computer and he said his game was lagging ... and he was mouthing off to her and she was mouthing off to him ... he actually left his Xbox and started physically attacking his sister and it

escalated to the point where, um, I had to call 911. And he kicks, he punches, and the thing that really, really worries me is he chokes.

LINDSAY [sibling/sister, 16 years old]: When he [brother] gets mad he just tantrums. He has punched my mum in her upper cheek area, and she, like, almost thought she broke it ... we've had to just leave the house until he calms down.

Turning to the literature, the aggression (physical and verbal) described by the caregivers and siblings is similar to other forms of family-based violence, such an intimate partner, sibling and/or domestic violence (Buckley, Holt, & Whelan, 2007; Eriksen & Jensen, 2009; Alhabib, Nur, & Jones, 2010; Button & Gealt, 2010; Renner, 2012).

The reactions family members had were also consistent with other forms of family-based violence.

GARY [sibling/brother, 21 years old]: You know, he'd just grab me or something, or choked me or something, or try to choke me, and start a fight or something, and ... one time ... he hit my mom and so I called the police on him, and – well, they said there was nothing they could do. My mom ... she was like ... 'oh, well. It wasn't a big deal' and was kind of undermining the whole issue.

NATASHA [sibling/sister, 14 years old]: Well, I just scared to be in the same room with him [brother] with any objects around me because even if it is a table, he'd pick it up and he'd literally throw it at me, he will hit me. Anything he can get his hands on basically, if I get him angry, he will hit me ... And I used to hide it from them [my parents] 'cause I didn't want my brother to leave me 'cause he's my only brother. So I used to cover his 'ass'.

HOLLY [mother]: [After being hit in the mouth with a metal water bottle by my daughter] I looked like I had a moustache. It wasn't good. And then I had to go to work the next day and explain what happened to my face. 'I was playing football with the kids...or baseball and the ball hit me'. ... Yeah, I mean I wasn't going to say ... I wouldn't want people to think that I'm, that, you know, there's a lot of violence in my house.

As a shame-based response, concealing the violence and injuries and/or minimising the severity of the violence are consistent with other forms of family-based violence where spouses, partners or children are concealing the abuse and injuries in order to demonstrate loyalty (Vandello et al., 2009), and to avoid shame as an experience of self-condemnation and having lost the respect of others (Mills, 2008; Enander, 2010; Stanley et al., 2012). These responses indicate the ways that self and family stigmas intersect in complex ways within families managing challenges related to a child's mental health. The experiences described, in particular by mother, Holly, of not wanting to reveal the challenges faced at home highlight the importance of centring interventions within a framework of understanding the stigma of mental and its potentially negative effects on individual family members, the family unit and helping-seeking.

As a practice-based consideration, of particular concern is that despite involvement with various child and youth mental health services, all the caregivers and siblings describe a lack of opportunity to adequately debrief their own experiences of distress related to the conflict, crisis and/or police encounters. The need for support is highlighted by Tim's experiences as a sibling.

> TIM [sibling/brother, 13 years old]: And that night that he [brother] went to the hospital [for an assessment because of threats of harm to himself], I mean, the police came and they took him away in handcuffs to the hospital and I was bawling my eyes out and it was, like, insane ... [After that night] honestly all I wanted to do, just to get it off my head, was talk about it. I just wanted to talk, like, just get it away, like, how my brother went there and just, like, just recalling the night just to try and ... Like, you know when you just saying, like, a word like ... you say it so much that you forget the meaning of it? I tried to say, talk about that so much just so I could get it out of my head ... Like, just the picture of him being taken away in handcuffs. I was just trying to get that out of my mind.

Tim draws attention not only to the distressing nature of the incident, but also to his distress of witnessing the police intervention with his brother. The intrusiveness of the imagery – Tim's reoccurring need after the event to talk repeatedly about his experiences in order to cope with the image of his brother being removed in handcuffs – was suggestive of a trauma reaction (Davis, 1999). Repeating the details of his brother's escort was Tim's attempt to diffuse the intensity of the emotional distress he experienced during the event, which continued after the event had ended (Silva, 2004).

A potential effect or outcome of family-based violence reported extensively in other areas is trauma, traumatisation and trauma-related reactions in children and caregivers (Fantuzzo & Mohr, 1999; Gorde et al., 2004; Silva, 2004; Spilsbury et al., 2007). Trauma refers to a psychological injury sustained related to witnessing or experiencing a traumatic event (Breslau, 2002; Wiger & Harowski, 2003) resulting in intense fear or helplessness (Yeager & Roberts, 2003; Jakovljevie, 2012). Considering the nature of the aggression (physical and/or verbal) described and the potential risks for trauma and traumatisation, the implementation of 'safety plans' similar to those used for other forms of family-based violence may be an important consideration for practice.

Depending on the particular form of family-based violence, safety plans have consisted of a range of practices, strategies and responses for making family environments safe/safer. For example, in child protection work, safety plans can consist of establishing and implementing practices aimed at changing parental behaviours (Gibson, 2014). For intimate partner violence, safety plans may include supporting women to assess the risks for harm (Campbell, 2004) and then having an action plan that would include knowing what to do and where to go when unsafe (Kendall et al., 2009). However, applying tools (such as safety plans) used for other forms of family-based violence to situations involving a person experiencing a psychiatric crisis requires special consideration. Safety plans imply a 'perpetrator' and a 'victim' and in mental health such constructions are problematic for reinforcing the stigma of mental illness. Viewing a distressed child as a 'perpetrator' of violence, and caregivers and siblings as 'victims' in need of protection reinforce and perpetuate prejudices that conceive mental illness with 'dangerousness'; a person living with a mental health issue as 'dangerous'; and persons associated with a person deemed mentally ill as vulnerable. The second main theme to emerge are the ways accessing police services for support is complicated by the stigma of mental illness, and in particular by encounters with family stigma.

Theme two: stigmatisation and criminalisation

Overall, caregivers and, especially, siblings describe police involvement as helpful for deescalating a high conflict situation, but as a mental health intervention, encounters with police are described as unhelpful. The main reason relates to the stigmatisation of the distressed child and their caregivers and siblings, as family members. The following narratives are examples of the main stigma experiences encountered by caregivers and siblings related to accessing police services.

> CHRISTINE [mother]: When the 'cops' are in [my son's] room there's a load of clean laundry in a laundry basket ... the police officers say, 'oh well, at least you've done his laundry'. Comments. Yeah, so that gets my back up ... don't judge a book by the cover. This cop has no idea what this family has gone through.
>
> RITA [mother]: I got woken up in the night because the police said that he'd been joy-riding and they had smashed ... And the police is really like, 'do you know where your kid is? Why don't you know where your kid is?' And meanwhile I'm in bed trying to get lots of sleep because I'm recovering from cancer treatment.
>
> NATASHA [sibling/sister, 14 years old]: It [the police intervention] was scary 'cause I didn't know what would happen to him [my brother]. There was a time where me and mom were at home, the time he pushed her down and we got into a huge fight – the whole family. My mom and I called the cops on him and he tried blaming the whole situation on us, and the cops obviously believed me and my mom because it's two against one and I'm laying there on the ground needing ambulance help.

These narratives tell a compelling story of the difficult predicament faced by caregivers and their children, who not only have to contend with the mental health issue but also with feeling or being judged negatively by responding officers.

The prejudices and discrimination associated with having a mental health issue are clearly articulated by mothers, Connie and Jeanette.

> CONNIE [mother]: What I have seen, that the police tend to take a different approach ... from a medical standpoint, they take it different. So it's two totally different approaches, two different strategies. It's two different worlds really. However, your kid gets caught in the middle. He might be in jail when he should have been in a hospital. And it's unfortunate because now he's labelled even more. Now he's got two things going for him – which is two negatives.
>
> JEANETTE [mother]: He [son, 12 years old] was walking home with three of the girls ... he tried to kiss the one girl because he actually liked her ... this girl didn't even report it. I guess the girl told her parents ... They didn't even call into the school to report it ... [the school] found out about this incident [from another student] so they called the community police officer and we got a call and [my son] had to be removed from school ... so then we had a big meeting ... with him [the police officer] and then he met with [our son] and he did a lot of talk about sexual assault and sexual harassment ... of course we shared everything, you know, [my son] as 'this and that' [about his issues] ... my husband then gets

a phone call [a few days later] saying that the officer reported back to the sergeant, they wanted to proceed with a police caution ... a formal document and it basically says that on or about this date, [my son] committed a sexual assault and we were asked to sign it and [my son] was asked to sign it .... I was just shocked that it got so far ... We thought it was just going to be a verbal warning ... but to take it to that level, I really felt that we were being judged because of his mental health ... what is happening to us and the trauma we're going through, it's just not right ... This is discrimination.

Inadvertently, police involvement can officially implicate the mental illness as dangerous or as potentially dangerous; the distressed young person as a potential criminal; caregivers and families as incompetent and culpable for failing in their parenting/caregiving roles; and family members as helpless and victims in need of protection from loved ones. The implications of this stigma for the child/youth, caregivers and siblings were serious, including being inappropriately treated within the criminal justice system rather than the mental health system, and exposure to the encounter as a traumatic event and as discrimination. As previously mentioned, the main issue with using police as a mental health intervention is that it contributes to the criminalisation of mental illness and of persons deemed to have a mental illness (Corrigan *et al.*, 2005; Gur, 2010; Chaimowitz, 2012). Given the nature of the crises that can occur the justification for police involvement is powerful; however, not without its own negative consequences, such as the criminalisation of the children and youth experiencing distress and the stigmatisation of caregivers and siblings, as family members.

It is important to note that among the caregivers who experienced police involvement for their child's mental health issue, there was one anomalous narrative that described police involvement as helpful and positive:

MARIE [mother]: We wanted her to go down to the hospital and she refused ... these two officers that came to the house were phenomenal. They sat up in her room on her bedroom floor for an hour and a half, talking to her. Got her calmed, got her to go to sleep .... we lucked in that night .... you could tell they really made a connection with teens and the mental health issues. They had some education on it, obviously, and it was phenomenal.

Similar to benefits noted in the literature, Marie suggests the factors that contributed to a positive encounter was the training the responding police officers appeared to have for working with children and youth (as a developmental stage unique from adulthood) and an awareness about mental health issues. Other benefits of CIT for police include: a reduction of stigmatising attitudes among police officers; a better understanding of mental health crisis and effective strategies for responding; and a sense of increased confidence and control over the situation (Demir *et al.*, 2009; Chopko, 2011; Canada *et al.*, 2012; Herrington & Pope, 2014).

Interestingly, parallel benefits are noted about parent education used to address a range of diverse issues: preventing child abuse and neglect, addressing child behaviours or learning about the effects of divorce. In particular, the benefits include: supporting parents to have more realistic expectations of their children; providing information about the effects of an issue on both the parents and child; providing practical strategies and skills to respond; and reducing isolation and building confidence (Atwood, 2000; Barth, 2009; Spielfogel *et al.*, 2011; To *et al.*, 2013). Given the complexity of the stigma faced by parents and their children, another benefit could be to provide and develop strategies for identifying and responding to the prejudices and discriminations encountered. Throughout parent education is cited as a promising approach for addressing a broad range of family-based concerns, and we concur that CIT for parents may also be viable model of support. In the next section, we discuss the implications of the outcomes for social work practice in child and youth mental health.

Implications for social work practice in child and youth mental health

Stigma-informed crisis intervention training for parents

There are two main implications that call for immediate consideration in social work practice in child and youth mental health. The first relates to the nature of the situations for which police can be involved with families, and the second is the stigma of mental illness. Family members are calling police services because they need support to deescalate a high conflict situation involving a distressed child/sibling. The nature of the conflict, which at times can include verbal and/or physical aggression, is serious; thus, the rationale for police involvement and safety planning are powerful. However, police involvement for mental health matters is not without consequences for the criminalisation of the child and youth experiencing mental health challenges and the stigmatisation of parents and siblings, as family members. As social workers, there is an important opportunity for combatting the stigma of mental illness and for supporting parents with planning responses that build safety and mitigate the risk for trauma. Given the benefits of parent education and of CIT for police, we propose a model of support that combines both – combatting stigma and supporting parental responses to crisis situations.

We suggest that CIT for parents could have similar benefits to those cited for police officer. Parent education can provide important information about mental health, child development, children's distress, crisis theory and interventions, as well as information about the stigma of mental illness as a structural condition of their personal experiences. By having information about the nature of 'mental illness' and of distress, caregivers can be supported to better understand their children's particular mental health issues and needs during moments of distress. For police officers, CIT contributed to shifts in negative views that mental health issues were a matter of personal and/or family misconduct resulting is a decrease of stigmatisation and stereotyping by responding officers (Demir *et al.*, 2009; Chopko, 2011). As a feature of family stigma, parents can have similar negative beliefs that their child's distress is intentional misbehaviour and/or defiance (Liegghio, 2013). Such beliefs may be problematic during times of conflict if parents respond by trying to discipline their children for what they understand to be misconduct rather than distress. Given the complex ways different forms of stigma intersect within the family as a unit and between the family and its contact with systems, such as the police, training informed by stigma will be important in order to support caregivers to develop strategies for recognising, responding, and combatting its potentially negative effects.

Second, caregivers can be supported to develop concrete skills, strategies, and tools for responding to their child's distress and family's needs, for example, by developing and implementing safety plans with an understanding of mitigating the potential for trauma. Considering the nature of the conflict, which at time includes violence, "safety plans" similar to those used for other forms of family-based violence may be an important tool. For police officers, CIT resulted in a better understanding of the child's distress, the risks and safety issues, and the responses for deescalating conflict (Canada et al., 2012). As an approach, training families on how to effectively respond to crisis and to make their family environments safe or safer may minimise and/or divert the involvement of police services for support.

Finally, stigma-informed CIT for parents could reduce isolation (Atwood, 2000) and strengthen their sense of confidence, competence and preparedness (Herrington & Pope, 2014). Building parental capacities and improving confidence can be important to countering the shame, self-blame and incompetence parents can feel or are made to feel as a feature of the family stigma they encounter (Liegghio, 2013). Like for police officers, having the skills necessary to respond more effectively to conflict and distress, parents may feel better prepared for maneuvering through a crisis using their own skills and knowledge to prevent and/or manage an escalation (Ritter et al., 2010). To conclude, considering the nature of the situations for which police are called for support, the stigma of mental illness and the potential benefits of parent education, CIT for parents informed by an understanding of the stigma of mental illness may be viable. Again, such training could provide caregivers with important support for identifying and responding to crisis and for developing family safety plans that may or may not involve police, but that could minimise and/or divert the need for their involvement. Thus, stigma-informed CIT for parents warrants serious consideration for social work practice in child and youth mental health and further research.

Acknowledgements

This work was supported by the Mental Health Commission of Canada.

Disclosure statement

No potential conflict of interest was reported by the authors.

Notes
1.   The terms 'caregiver' and 'parents' will be used interchangeably to refer to all childrearing arrangements, including biological, step, adoptive and foster parents, as well as grandparents and/or kinship relatives.
2.   For a complete discussion of the stigma of mental illness in child and youth mental health, refer to Liegghio, 2013.

3.   When we factor in the experiences of all 29 participants, including the perspectives of the seven youth-participants, the rate of involvement with police increases to 63%.

References

Alhabib, S., Nur, U. & Jones, R. (2010, May) 'Domestic violence against women: systematic review of prevalence studies', *Journal of Family Violence*, vol. 25, no. 4, pp. 369–382.

Atwood, J. (2000) 'The family therapist in the courts', *Journal of Prevention and Intervention in the Community*, vol. 21, no. 1, pp. 113–124. doi:10.1300/J005v21n01_08.

Barth, R. (2009) 'Preventing child abuse and neglect with parent training: evidence and opportunities', *The Future of Children*, vol. 19, no. 2, pp. 95–118. doi:10.1353/foc. 0.0031.

Boyle, M. & Willms, J. D. (2002) 'Impact evaluation of a national, community-based program for at-risk children in Canada', *Canadian Public Policy*, vol. 28, no. 3, pp. 461–481. doi:10.2307/3552232.

Braidwood Commission (2009, June 18) *Restoring Public Confidence: Restricting the Use of Conducted Energy Weapons in British Columbia*, Braidwood Commission on Conducted Energy Weapons, Victoria, British Columbia, Retrieved on June 4, 2014, from http://www.braidwoodinquiry.ca/report

Breslau, E. (2002) 'Epidemiologic studies of trauma, posttraumatic stress disorder, and other psychiatric disorders', *Canadian Journal of Psychiatry*, vol. 47, no. 10, pp. 923–930.

Brink, J., Livingston, J., Desmarais, S., Greaves, C., Maxwell, V., Michalak, E., Parent, R., Verdun-Jones, S. & Weaver, C. (2011) *A Study of How People with Mental Illness Perceive and Interact with the Police*, Mental Health Commission of Canada, Calgary, Alberta, Retrieved on October 2, 2013, from http://www.mentalhealthcommission

Burnard (1991) 'A method of analysing interview transcripts in qualitative research', *Nurse Education Today*, vol. 11, pp. 23–37.

Buckley, H., Holt, S. & Whelan, S. (2007, September) 'Listen to me! Children's experiences of domestic violence', *Child Abuse Review*, vol. 16, no. 5, pp. 296–310.

Button, D. & Gealt, R. (2010) 'High risk behaviors among victims of sibling violence', *Journal of Family Violence*, vol. 25, pp. 131–140.

Campbell, J. (2004) 'Helping women understand their risk in situations of intimate partner violence', *Journal of Interpersonal Violence*, vol. 19, no. 12, pp. 1464–1477. doi:10. 1177/0886260504269698.

Canada, K., Angell, B. & Watson, A. (2012) 'Intervening at the entry point: differences in how CIT trained and non-CIT trained officers describe responding to mental health-related calls', *Journal of Community Mental Health*, vol. 48, no. 6, pp. 746–755. doi:10.1007/s10597-011-9430-9.

Carswell, K., Maughan, B., Davis, H., Davenport, F. & Goddard, N. (2004) 'The psychosocial needs of young offenders and adolescents from an inner city area', *Journal of Adolescence*, vol. 27, no. 4, pp. 415–428. doi:10.1016/j.adolescence.2004. 04.003.

Chaimowitz, G. (2012, February) 'The criminalization of people with mental illness', *Canadian Journal of Psychiatry*, vol. 57, no. 2, pp. 1–7.

Chammartin, N., Ogaranko, C. & Froese, B. (2011) *Equality, Dignity and Inclusion: Legislation that Enhances Human Rights for People Living with Mental Illness*, Mental Health Commission of Canada, Calgary, Alberta, Retrieved on October 2, 2013, from http://www.mentalhealthcommission

Chassin, L. (2008, Fall) 'Juvenile justice and substance use', *The Future of Children*, vol. 18, no. 2, pp. 165–183. doi:10.1353/foc.0.0017.

Chopko, B. A. (2011) 'Walk in balance: training crisis intervention team police officers as compassionate warriors', *Journal of Creativity in Mental Health*, vol. 6, no. 4, pp. 315–328. doi:10.1080/15401383.2011.630304.

Coleman, T. & Cotton, D. (2010) *Interactions with Persons with a Mental Illness: Police Learning in the Environment of Contemporary Policing*, Mental Health Commission of Canada, Calgary, Alberta, Retrieved on October 2, 2013, from www.mentalhealthcommission

Coleman, T. & Cotton, D. (2014) *TEMPO: Police Interactions – A Report Towards Improving Interactions Between Police and People Living with Mental Health Problems*, Mental Health Commission of Canada, Calgary, Alberta, Retrieved on September 30, 2014, from www.mentalhealthcommission

Corrigan, P., Watson, A., Byrne, P. & Davis, K. (2005, October) 'Mental illness stigma: problem of public health or social justice?', *Social Work*, vol. 50, no. 4, pp. 363–368. doi:10.1093/sw/50.4.363.

Coleman, T. & Cotton, D. (2010) *Police Interactions with Persons with a Mental Illness: Police Learning in an Environment of Contemporary Policing*, Mental Health Commission of Canada, Calgary, Alberta, Retrieved on July 4, 2014, from www.mentalhealthcommission.ca/English/system/files/private/Law_Police_Interactions_Mental_Illness_Report_ENG_0.pdf?terminitial=24

Cotton, D. & Coleman, T. (2008) *A Study of Police Academy Training and Evaluation for New Police Officers Related to Working with People with Mental Illness*, Mental Health Commission of Canada, Calgary, Alberta, Retrieved on October 2, 2013, from http://www.mentalhealthcommission

Creswell, J. (1998) 'Five different qualitative studies', in *Qualitative Inquiry and Research Design*, Sage, Thousand Oaks, CA, pp. 27–72.

Davis, H. (1999, October) 'The psychiatrization of post-traumatic distress: issues for social workers', *British Journal of Social Work*, vol. 29, no. 5, pp. 755–777. doi:10.1093/bjsw/29.5.755.

Demir, B., Broussard, B., Goulding, S. M. & Compton, M. T. (2009) 'Beliefs about causes of schizophrenia among police officers before and after crisis intervention team training', *Community Mental Health Journal*, vol. 45, no. 5, pp. 385–392. doi:10.1007/s10597-009-9194-7.

Doulas, A. & Lurigio, D. (2010) 'Youth crisis intervention teams (CITs): a response to the fragmentation of the educational, mental health, and juvenile justice systems', *Journal of Police Crisis Negotiations*, vol. 10, nos. 1–2, pp. 241–263. doi:10.1080/15332586.2010.481893.

Eden, D. (2014) *Verdict Explanation: Inquest into the Deaths of Reyal Jardine-Douglas, Sylvia Klibingaitis and Michael Elgin Jr*, Office of the Chief Coroner, Toronto, Ontario, Retrieved from http://www.mcscs.jus.gov.on.ca/english/DeathInvestigations/office_coroner/PublicationsandReports/OCC_pubs.html

Enander, V. (2010, January) '"A fool to keep staying": battered women labeling themselves stupid as an expression of gendered shame', *Violence Against Women*, vol. 16, no. 1, pp. 5–31. doi:10.1177/1077801209353577.

Erickson, P. & Butters, J. (2005) 'How does the Canadian juvenile justice system respond to detained youth with substance use associated problems? Gaps, challenges, and emerging issues', *Substance Use and Misuse*, vol. 40, no. 7, pp. 953–973. doi:10.1081/JA-200058855.

Eriksen, S. & Jensen, V. (2009) 'A push or a punch: distinguishing the severity of sibling violence', *Journal of Interpersonal Violence*, vol. 24, no. 1, pp. 183–208. doi:10.1177/0886260508316298.

Fantuzzo, J. & Mohr, W. (1999, January) 'Prevalence and effects of child exposure to domestic violence', *Future of Children*, vol. 9, no. 3, pp. 21–32. doi:10.2307/1602779.

Fry, A., O'Riordan, D. & Geanellos, R. (2002, July) 'Social control agents or front-line carers for people with mental health problems: police and mental health services in Sydney, Australia', *Health and Social Care in the Community*, vol. 10, no. 4, pp. 277–286. doi:10.1046/j.1365-2524.2002.00371.x.

Gibson, M. (2014) 'Narrative practice and the signs of safety approach: engaging adolescents in building rigorous safety plans', *Child in Care Practice*, vol. 20, no. 1, pp. 64–80. doi:10.1080/13575279.2013.799455.

Gorde, M., Helfrich, C. & Finlayson, M. (2004, June) 'Trauma symptoms and life skill needs of domestic violence victims', *Journal of Interpersonal Violence*, vol. 19, no. 6, pp. 691–708. doi:10.1177/0886260504263871.

Gur, O. (2010, June) 'Persons with mental illness in the criminal justice system: police interventions prevent violence and criminalization', *Journal of Police Crisis Negotiations*, vol. 10, nos. 1–2, pp. 220–240.

Hinshaw, S. (2005) 'The stigmatization of mental illness in children and parents: developmental issues, family concerns, and research needs', *Journal of Child Psychology & Psychiatry*, vol. 46, no. 7, pp. 714–734. doi:10.1111/j.1469-7610.2005.01456.x.

Herrington, V. & Pope, R. (2014) 'The impact of police training in mental health: an example from Australia', *Policing and Society*, vol. 24, no. 5, pp. 501–522. doi:10.1080/10439463.2013.784287.

Iacobucci, F. (2014, July) *Police Encounters with People in Crisis* (An independent review conducted by the Honourable Frank Iacobucci for the Chief of Police, William Blair, Toronto Police Service, Toronto, Ontario). Retrieved on August 12, 2014, from http://www.tpsreview.ca/docs/Police-Encounters-With-People-In-Crisis.pdf

Jakovljevie, M. (2012) 'Posttraumatic stress disorder (PTSD): a tailor-made diagnosis for an age of disenchantment and disillusionment?', *Psychiatria Danubina*, vol. 24, no. 3, pp. 238–240.

Kendall, J., Pelucio, M., Casaletto, J., Thompson, K., Barnes, S., Pettit, E. & Aldrich, M. (2009, February) 'Impact of emergency department intimate partner violence intervention', *Journal of Interpersonal Violence*, vol. 24, no. 2, pp. 280–306. doi:10.1177/0886260508316480.

Kirby, M. & Keon, W. J. (2006, May) *Out of the Shadows at Last: Transforming Mental Health, Mental Illness and Addictions Services in Canada*, Government of Canada, The Standing Senate Committee on Social Affairs, Science and Technology, Ottawa, Ontario.

Koro-Ljungberg, M. & Bussing, R. (2009) 'The management of courtesy stigma in the lives of families with teenagers with ADHD', *Journal of Family Issues*, vol. 30, no. 9, pp. 1175–1200. doi:10.1177/0192513X09333707.

Kress, V., Adamson, N., Paylo, M., DeMarco, C. & Bradley, N. (2012) 'The use of safety plans with children and adolescents living in violence homes', *The Family Journal: Counseling and Therapy for Couples and Families*, vol. 20, no. 3, pp. 249–255.

Liegghio, M. (2013) 'The stigma of mental illness: learning from the situated knowledge of psychiatrized youth, caregivers and young siblings', (Doctoral thesis, Faculty of Social Work, Wilfrid Laurier University).

Liegghio, M., Van Katwyk, T., Freeman, B., Caragata, L., Sdao-Jarvie, K., Brown, K. C. & Sandu, A. Policing and police encounters among a community population of children and youth accessing mental health services (in press).

Mills, L. (2008, June) Shame and intimate abuse: the critical missing link between cause and cure. *Children and Youth Services Review*, vol. 30, no. 6, pp. 631–638.

Morabito, M., Kerr, A., Watson, A., Draine, J., Ottati, V. & Angell, B. (2012) 'Crisis intervention teams and people with mental illness: exploring the factors that influence the use of force', *Crime & Delinquency*, vol. 58, no. 1, pp. 57–77. doi:10.1177/0011128710372456.

Moskos, M., Olson, L., Halbern, S. & Gray, D. (2007, April) 'Utah youth suicide study: barriers to mental health treatment for adolescents', *Suicide and Life-Threatening Behavior*, vol. 37, no. 2, pp. 179–186. doi:10.1521/suli.2007.37.2.179.

Munson, M., Floersch, J. & Townsend, L. (2009) 'Attitudes toward mental health services and illness perceptions among adolescents with mood disorders', *Child and Adolescent Social Work Journal*, vol. 26, no. 5, pp. 447–466. doi:10.1007/s10560-009-0174-0.

Odgers, C., Burnette, M., Chauhan, P., Moretti, M. & Reppucci, D. (2005) 'Misdiagnosing the problem: mental health profiles of incarcerated juveniles', *The Canadian Child and Adolescent Psychiatry Review*, vol. 14, no. 1, pp. 26–29.

Offord, D., Chmura-Kraemer, H., Kazdin, A., Jensen, P. & Harrington, R. (1998, July) 'Lowering the burden of suffering from child psychiatric disorder: trade-offs among clinical, targeted, and universal interventions', *Journal of the American Academy of Child and Adolescent Psychiatry*, vol. 37, no. 7, pp. 686–694.

O'Reilly, M., Taylor, H. & Vostanis, P. (2009) '"Nuts, schiz, psycho": an exploration of young homeless people's perceptions and dilemmas of defining mental health', *Social Science & Medicine*, vol. 68, no. 9, pp. 1737–1744. doi:10.1016/j.socscimed.2009.02.033.

Renner, L. (2012, April) 'Single types of family violence victimization and externalizing behaviors among children and adolescents', *Journal of Family Violence*, vol. 27, no.3, pp. 177–186.

Richardson, L. (2001) 'Seeking and obtaining mental health services: what do parents expect?', *Archives of Psychiatric Nursing*, vol. 15, no. 5, pp. 223–231. doi:10.1053/apnu.2001.27019.

Ritter, C., Teller, J., Munetz, M. & Bonfine, N. (2010) 'Crisis intervention team (CIT) training: selection effects and long-term changes in perceptions of mental illness and community preparedness', *Journal of Police Crisis Negotiations*, vol. 10, nos. 1–2, pp. 133–152.

Robst, J., Armstrong, M., Dollard, N. & Rohrer, L. (2013) 'Arrests among youth after out-of-home mental health treatment: comparisons across community and residential treatment settings', *Criminal Behavior and Mental Health*, vol. 23, no. 3, pp. 162–176. doi:10.1002/cbm.1871.

Samargia, L., Saewyc, E. & Elliott, B. (2006, February) 'Foregone mental health care and self-reported access barriers among adolescents', *Journal of School Nursing*, vol. 22, no. 1, pp. 17–24. doi:10.1177/10598405060220010401.

Shanley, D., Reid, G. & Evans, B. (2008) 'How parents seek help for children with mental health problems', *Administration and Policy in Mental Health and Mental Health Services Research*, vol. 35, no. 3, pp. 135–146. doi:10.1007/s10488-006-0107-6.

Silk, J., Nath, S., Siegel, L. & Kendall, P. (2000) 'Conceptualizing mental disorders in children: where have we been and where are we going?', *Development and Psychopathology*, vol. 12, no. 4, pp. 713–735. doi:10.1017/S0954579400004090.

Silva, R. (2004) *Posttraumatic Stress Disorders in Children and Adolescents*, W.W. Norton & Company, New York.

Spielfogel, J., Leathers, S., Christian, E. & McMeel, L. (2011) 'Parent management training, relationships with agency staff, and child mental health: urban foster parents' perspectives', *Children and Youth Services Review*, vol. 33, no. 11, pp. 2366–2374. doi:10.1016/j.childyouth.2011.08.008.

Spilsbury, J., Belliston, L., Drotar, D., Drinkard, A., Kretschmar, J., Creeden, R., Flannery, D. & Friedman, S. (2007) 'Clinically significant trauma symptoms and behavioral problems in a community-based sample of children exposed to domestic violence', *Journal of Family Violence*, vol. 22, no. 6, pp. 487–499. doi:10.1007/s10896-007-9113-z.

Stanley, N., Miller, P. & Richardson Foster, H. (2012) 'Engaging with children's and parents' perspectives on domestic violence', *Child & Family Social Work*, vol. 17, no. 2, pp. 192–201. doi:10.1111/j.1365-2206.2012.00832.x.

Strauss, A. & Corbin, J. (1998) *Basics of Qualitative Research: Techniques and Procedures for Developing Grounded Theory*. 2nd ed. Sage, Thousand Oaks, CA.

To, S., Iu kan, S., Tsoi, K. & Chan, T. (2013) 'A qualitative analysis of parents' perceived outcomes and experiences in a parent education program adopting a transformative approach', *Journal of Social Work Practice*, vol. 27, no. 1, pp. 79–94. doi:10.1080/02650533.2012.732046.

Townsend, E., Walker, D., Sargeant, S., Vostanis, P., Hawton, K., Stocker, O. & Sithole, J. (2010) 'Systematic review and meta-analysis of interventions relevant for young offenders with mood disorders, anxiety disorders, or self-harm', *Journal of Adolescence*, vol. 33, no. 1, pp. 9–20. doi:10.1016/j.adolescence.2009.05.015.

Tuchman, G. (1996) 'ESS presidential address, 1995 – invisible differences: on the management of children in postindustrial society', *Sociological Forum*, vol. 11, no. 1, pp. 3–23. doi:10.1007/BF02408299.

Vandello, J., Cohen, D., Grandon, R. & Franiuk, R. (2009, January) 'Stand by your man: indirect prescriptions for honorable violence and feminine loyalty in Canada, Chile, and the United States', *Journal of Cross-Cultural Psychology*, vol. 40, no. 1, pp. 81–104. doi:10.1177/0022022108326194.

Vander Koep, A., Evens, C. & Taub, J. (1997) 'I. Risk of juvenile justice system referral among children in a public mental health system', *Journal of Behavioral Health Sciences and Research*, vol. 24, no. 4, pp. 428–442. doi:10.1007/BF02790504.

Watson, A., Angell, B., Morabito, M. & Robinson, N. (2008, November) 'Defying negative expectations: dimensions of fair and respectful treatment by police officers as perceived by people with mental illness', *Administration and Policy in Mental Health* and *Mental Health Services Research*, vol. 35, no. 6, pp. 449–457. doi:10.1007/s10488-008-0188-5.

Wiger, D. & Harowski, K. (2003) *Essentials of Crisis Counselling and Intervention*, Wiley, Hoboken, NJ.

Yeager, K. & Roberts, A. (2003, March) 'Differentiating among stress, acute stress disorder, crisis episodes, trauma, and PTSD: paradigm and treatment goals', *Brief Treatment and Crisis Intervention*, vol. 3, no. 1, pp. 3–26. doi:10.1093/brief-treatment/mhg002.

Zimmerman, F. (2005) 'Social and economic determinants of disparities in professional help-seeking for child mental health problems: evidence from a national sample', *Health Research and Educational Trust*, vol. 40, no. 5, pp. 1514–1533.

Marika Morris and Claire Crooks

STRUCTURAL AND CULTURAL FACTORS IN SUICIDE PREVENTION: THE CONTRAST BETWEEN MAINSTREAM AND INUIT APPROACHES TO UNDERSTANDING AND PREVENTING SUICIDE

This article is a documentary analysis of Inuit knowledge about suicide prevention which yields insights into how structural and cultural factors are essential to curbing suicide in marginalized populations. This study investigated the grey literature produced by Inuit community organizations and Inuit-led regional governments for Inuit understandings of suicide, its causes and prevention. Findings include that Inuit identify rapid colonization and its effects as the root of Inuit's highest suicide rate of any group in Canada; that suicide cannot be viewed in isolation from socio-economic conditions; that restoring the cultural pride of Inuit is essential to mental well-being; and that Inuit have created suicide prevention models building on strengths, relationship skills building and engaging the community, particularly youth and elders. This article makes an important contribution to the academic literature and social work practice in documenting Inuit suicide prevention concepts as a complement to western models which focus on individual depression.

Introduction

Inuit have one of the highest suicide rates in the world (Health Canada, 2006). Yet, a culturally competent understanding of this phenomenon remains absent from most prevention literature and training materials. Comprehending suicide among Inuit requires an understanding of both structural and cultural factors. This article explores Inuit suicide prevention concepts in an effort to encourage social work faculties and professional bodies to recognize the importance of structural factors and cultural knowledge in marginalized populations when designing suicide prevention curricula for students or practising professionals, rather than limiting themselves to the mainstream focus on individual depression. Several studies have pointed out that social workers are likely to encounter clients at risk for suicide, but most receive no training or insufficient training, education or other preparation to deal effectively to engage in suicide prevention (Jacobson *et al.*, 2012; Ruth *et al.*, 2012; Osteen *et al.*, 2014; Scott, 2015). In the context of the growing call for social work researchers, professionals and faculties to address suicide (Scott, 2015), cultural competency in suicide prevention is also important (Hamilton & Rolf, 2010).

Inuit are the most recently colonized of all Indigenous peoples in Canada. Within living memory, Inuit experienced self-sufficiency and self-governance before Canadian government actions of the 1940s to 1960s to control the Canadian Arctic. The assertion by Inuit elders that suicide was rare among Inuit before colonization is buttressed by some early academic work that suicide among Inuit in 1935 was very low, an estimated 3.0 per 100,000 (Hicks, 2007). Kirmayer *et al.* (1998) also asserted that suicide in precolonial Inuit societies was a rare event that mainly involved some elderly, ill or disabled Inuit taking their lives during times of famine. Hicks (2007) pointed out that rising Inuit suicide rates in various regions in Canada and the circumpolar world correspond to when that region was actively colonized by *Qallunaat* (white people), with the highest suicide rates emerging one generation later.

Canada's Chief Public Health Officer reported that suicide rates in regions in which Inuit live are now 11 times as high as in the general Canadian population (PHAC, 2012). The suicide rate among youth is even more dramatic. Oliver *et al.* (2012, p. 4) documented that '[i]n 2004–2008, children and teenagers in Inuit Nunangat [regions in which Inuit live] were more than 30 times as likely to die from suicide as were those in the rest of Canada'. Inuit youth suicide rates are among the highest in the world, and higher than any other Indigenous group in Canada (Health Canada, 2006).

Colonization of Inuit was characterized by life-changing trauma. The Government of Canada acknowledged that its residential school policy deliberately tried to erase Indigenous cultures, languages, spiritual beliefs and traditions, and that it served to break the bonds between child and parents, community and culture (Harper, 2008). Children were separated by law from their parents, and sent to become 'civilized' at these schools, where many endured physical and sexual abuse. When they emerged, they did not have the skills, knowledge or motivation to live a traditional life, never developed parenting skills, nor did they have sufficient skills or were accepted enough by non-Indigenous society to integrate into the non-Indigenous economy (Royal Commission on Aboriginal Peoples, 1996).

The unresolved physical and sexual abuse endured at these schools became intergenerational. The 2007–2008 Inuit Health Survey in Nunavut (Galloway & Saudny, 2012) found that 31% of respondents experienced severe physical abuse as children, and 52% of women and 22% of men reported having experienced severe sexual abuse during childhood. We know that sustained experiences of physical and sexual abuse are strongly related to completed suicide attempts (Jokinen *et al.*, 2010).

Inuit are culturally and historically distinct from First Nations and Metis, the other Indigenous groups recognized in the Canadian Constitution. Inuit and First Nations share the history of residential schools, except that Inuit make up a disproportionate number of existing residential school survivors as the residential schools in the North were among the last to close (Weber, 2012). Inuit and First Nations also share a history of forced relocation, but it is within living memory that Inuit were forced to settle, had children and youth removed, had traditional economic pursuits limited or destroyed and were forced to live under the governance of strangers of another race, culture and language (Royal Commission on Aboriginal Peoples, 1996):

> ... the violence and abuse [in our communities] can be tracked back to two main causes: uncontrollable changes to culture and tradition; and feelings of loss of control over the future. These can lead to mental trauma, the breakdown of families, alcohol and drug addictions and feelings of powerlessness. Fear, mistrust, abuse and denial result, creating a cycle of abuse in which Inuit can be both victims and abusers – a cycle that repeats itself with each new generation. (Pauktuutit Inuit Women of Canada, 2007, p. 4)

In their research on Inuit suicide, Tester and McNicoll (2004, p. 2625) conclude 'that examining colonial relations of ruling, intersecting with the autonomy afforded Inuit youth, is essential to understanding the contemporary problem of young Inuit suicide'. Previous academic articles about Inuit conceptions of suicide and its prevention were very useful, small-scale qualitative studies of individuals in one location (e.g. Tester & McNicoll, 2004; Wexler *et al.*, 2013). This article is an analysis of Inuit community documentation related to Inuit suicide prevention, focusing on reports of consultations of Inuit across broad areas, and perspectives of Inuit service providers and leaders. Inuit have expressed the need for professionals who work with them to be more culturally aware (Inungni Sapujjijiit Task Force on Suicide Prevention and Community Healing, 2003; Alianait Inuit-specific Mental Wellness Task Group, 2007). This awareness is of course important for social workers who move to the Canadian North, but increasingly for all Canadian social workers as 25% of Inuit now living outside the Inuit Nunangat (traditional Inuit lands), many in large Canadian cities (Statistics Canada, 2013). Inuit also live in three other countries: Inuit/Inupiat/Yupik traditional lands stretch from Siberia (Russia), across Alaska (USA), Canada and Greenland (Denmark). Beyond better serving the Inuit population, this analysis brings Inuit knowledge of suicide and suicide prevention to the academic literature as an example of an Indigenous group identifying structural and cultural factors as important elements of suicide prevention interventions.

Method

This study is a documentary analysis which identified and reviewed Inuit grey literature – publications, statements and audiovisual resources by Inuit organizations and the Government of Nunavut – related in whole or in part to suicide and its prevention. Inuit have an oral culture, and therefore audiovisual documentation is important to include (Carry *et al.*, 2011). All materials will nonetheless be referred to in this article as the 'Inuit suicide prevention literature'.

Seventeen source materials from eight Inuit organizations and governments were identified as presenting an Inuit-specific approach to suicide prevention. Inclusion criteria were: the literature had to be generated by an Inuk,[1] Inuit organization or Inuit government; the work was based on widespread community consultation with Inuit over large geographical areas *or* was a summary of knowledge by Inuit healers and leaders *or* was material developed to be used in connection with Inuit suicide prevention. The following lists the literature used in this analysis:

1. Inuit Tapiriit Kanatami (ITK), founded in 1971 as the national organization representing Inuit in Canada.

   a. *Alianait Inuit Mental Wellness Action Plan:* The Alianait Inuit-specific Mental Wellness Task Group 'was mandated to create an Inuit-specific national strategy that reflects Inuit mental wellness priorities and circumstances' (2007, p. 1).
   b. National Inuit Leader Terry Audla's speech on World Suicide Prevention Day (Audla, 2013).

2. Pauktuutit Inuit Women of Canada, the national voice for Inuit women in Canada.

   a. *Inuit Healing in Contemporary Inuit Society* (2004): report of research in which 22 Inuit healers and elders were interviewed.
   b. *Making Our Shelters Strong: Training for Inuit Shelter Workers Participant Handbook* (2007): This manual for workers in shelters for abuse Inuit women and their children contains a segment on suicide prevention.

3. National Inuit Youth Council (NIYC), founded in 1994 to represent the concerns of Inuit youth. In 2002, NIYC made suicide prevention one of its top priorities.

   a. NIYC Celebration of Life statement in 2012.
   b. NIYC Celebration of Life statement in 2010.

4. Ajunnginiq Centre/Inuit Tuttarvingat, the Inuit-specific centre of the National Aboriginal Health Organization (NAHO), an Aboriginal-designed and Aboriginal-controlled body committed to influencing and advancing the health and well-being of Aboriginal peoples by carrying out knowledge-based strategies.

   a. Suicide prevention: Inuit traditional practices that encouraged resilience and coping (Korhonen, 2006).
   b. Resilience: Overcoming challenges and moving on positively (Korhonen, 2007).
   c. 'How are we as men?' – an interactive television programme and DVD in the three-part series *Qanuqtuurniq – Finding the Balance*, first aired in 2009. This episode of the programme is about Inuit men's health and well-being, and includes 13 mentions of suicide.
   d. 'I am young and I am proud', part of the *Qanuqtuurniq – Finding the Balance* series. This episode is about youth well-being, with a significant component devoted to suicide prevention.

5. Tungasuvvingat Inuit (TI), an Ottawa-based Inuit social service agency. The proceedings of the *Mamisarniq Conference 2007 Inuit-specific Approaches to Healing from Addiction and Trauma* also addresses suicide.
6. Blueprint for Life, an organization which produced a 2013 video documenting their 'Social Work for Hip Hop' workshop and subsequent hip hop programme which developed in Clyde River, Nunavut, which seeks to promote youth wellness and prevent suicide.
7. Kamatsiaqtut Help Line, a telephone helpline for people in Nunavut and Nunavik (northern Quebec). A Kamatsiaqtut brochure was included in this analysis.
8. Government of Nunavut.

a. *Our Words Must Come Back to Us*, the 2003 report of the Inungni Sapujjijiit Task Force on Suicide Prevention and Community Healing, which met with people in 17 Inuit communities.

b. *Towards the Development of a Nunavut Suicide Prevention Strategy: A Summary Report of the 2009 Community Consultations* (Government of Nunavut, 2009): the 2009 community consultations involved 525 participants through group meetings, radio call-in shows, community discussions and other methods of communication.

c. *Nunavut Suicide Prevention Strategy Action Plan* (Government of Nunavut, 2011): the Government of Nunavut partnered with Nunavut Tunngavik, the Isaksimagit Inuusirmi Katujjiqaatigiit Embrace Life Council and the Royal Canadian Mounted Police (RCMP) to create the Nunavut Suicide Prevention Strategy (2010) and Action Plan (2011).

A first pass-through the material was performed to identify general themes related to explanations of suicide, conceptions of suicide prevention and efforts to prevent suicide. A matrix was developed and a second, systematic pass-through was conducted to categorize statements in the 17 pieces of literature into identified themes. Where the literature was broader than suicide, only the parts that specifically addressed suicide or where the statements were clearly meant to apply to suicide were categorized. The themes were distilled into those on which the most consensus was achieved, which resulted in the final nine reported below. The results are presented in synthesis form rather than outlining what every piece stated about each topic. However, illustrative quotes are used to respect what Inuit told the Inungni Sapujjijiit Task Force on Suicide Prevention and Community Healing (2003), that researchers and governments parachute in to talk to them, but that their actual words are not reflected in the reports. Our aim was to produce a descriptive rather than critical analysis, as when Inuit experience is reported at all, it is usually viewed through a western cultural lens.

Results and analysis

Few peoples have experienced the incidence of suicide and suicide-related trauma than ... Inuit have. (Government of Nunavut, 2011)

The Inuit suicide prevention literature is unanimous in ascribing the rise in Inuit suicide rates to recent and rapid colonialization and its continued effects. In addition to the need for more mental health services, it also presents a holistic vision of mental wellness and suicide prevention that includes socio-economic and cultural wellness. Developing a positive cultural identity is seen as a central component of suicide prevention, as well as addressing the continuing effects of colonialization, such as hopelessness, addictions and violence. Suicide prevention outreach that takes a positive approach, in terms of building resilience, providing youth with something positive and healthy to do, teaching skills such as traditional skills, parenting and relationship skills, and providing space for people to speak out are the preferred approaches. The literature stresses the involvement of elders, youth and the community in suicide prevention strategies and activities, including suicide intervention training for community members. The need for Inuit-specific and Inuit-controlled services was also key. This section discusses these findings.

Many problems, same roots

One of the most devastating aspects of colonialization was the policy to separate Indigenous children from their parents and communities and send them to residential schools designed to erase their culture, language and spiritual beliefs. A survivor described the experience:

> ... at a very early age I was abused, sexually and physically. They took away all of our clothes, all of our belongings and they shaved our heads. They took away our names, our identity, gave us a number. I remember going to bed at night in our bunks and laying there crying because I was all alone. There was nobody there to hold me, to tell me I was alright. It was painful being brought up that way. Being beaten for things you didn't understand. And somehow survive it. And you bury it, hide it so that nobody ever sees it. (Inuit Tuttarvingat, 2009a, p. 16)

Beyond residential schools, Canadian government actions had an impact on the traditional Inuit economy and social roles. One such action was the killing of Inuit sled dogs, which were the only means of transportation and hunting, in the 1950s and 1960s. This had a profound negative effect on the role of Inuit men as hunters and providers (Inuit Tuttarvingat, 2009a). One of the things elders remember from life before colonization was that everyone was busy and knew their roles (Inuit Tuttarvingat, 2009b). Now for many Inuit, there is nothing productive to do.

Although Inuit have worked hard and succeeded in some areas in regaining control of their own governance, health and education systems, colonialization is still ongoing and Inuit are still overwhelmed with values not their own:

> Euro-Canadian values are at odds with Inuit values. For example, Euro-Canadian values stress [being] better, getting more game, winning, not sharing, these kinds of values [are ones] that can't work in Inuit culture. And you know, television and media have been introduced in our communities for quite some time now and they stress those very things. (Inuit Tuttarvingat, 2009a, p. 6)

Colonization is not something that happened in the past, it is ongoing, and continues to cause problems when the results of the damage done to Inuit are dealt with using western methods. The general suicide prevention literature does not tend to discuss corrections contexts, unless the work is specifically about suicide prevention in correctional facilities. Some of the Inuit literature mentions incarceration and its impact on mental wellness. One Inuit elder believed that at least half of Inuit men have been incarcerated at some time from the 1970s to today, and that incarceration had a negative impact on them (Inuit Tuttarvingat, 2009a). The dominant method used by the Government of Canada to deal with violence in Inuit communities is to put perpetrators in jail, usually very far from home. Inuit healers noted that perpetrators have almost always themselves been victims of child sexual, physical and emotional abuse (Pauktuutit Inuit Women of Canada, 2004). Inungni Sapujjijiit Task Force on Suicide Prevention and Community Healing (2003) points to interaction with the justice and correctional systems as suicide risk factors, even when awaiting a court date or sentencing, or after having come home.

Despite the challenges on so many fronts, Inuit visions for the future remain positive (Audla, 2013). Inuit are trying to forge an identity as Inuit in the modern world, create economic opportunities, heal from the pain of colonialization and abuse and help other Inuit resist suicide.

A vision of wellness beyond treating symptoms

The literature envisions holistic views of mental wellness, suicide prevention and preventing substance abuse that incorporate housing, economic development and jobs as key actions, in addition to regaining cultural pride.

The *Alianait Inuit Mental Wellness Action Plan* specified the following goals for mental health and suicide prevention:

> Inuit will have: ample opportunities for positive self-expression; the best of contemporary and traditional ways of life and the life skills to thrive in their environment; and socio-economic conditions that promote mental wellness. Ultimately, Inuit will live in a society in which each person has a valued purpose and role and is a contributing and necessary member of the community. (Alianait Inuit-specific Mental Wellness Task Group, 2007, p. 11)

Developing a positive and knowledgeable cultural identity

> We live in a time now where people have different types of expectations … We are going toward a Qallunaq [white people's] way of life. Suicide is the result of the lack of identity, loss of pride, fear of failure. (Government of Nunavut, 2009, p. 12)

Inuit youth, in particular, are caught between two cultures. On the one hand, developing a positive cultural identity, feeling connected to family, community and the land, is an important component of mental wellness. On the other hand, being able to negotiate the modern world and economy in a foreign language (English or French) is also important for socio-economic well-being. Inuit youth are faced with the challenge of how to be Inuit in rapidly changing world. Using Inuit cultural knowledge was one of the common characteristics of Inuit approaches to healing. Being proud of being Inuit and learning Inuit values were seen as important to suicide prevention.

Building resilience to be able to deal with challenges

Resilience is defined in the Inuit literature as 'the ability to keep, regain and build hope, emotional wellness, and positive ways of coping through times of difficulties in life' (Alianait Inuit-specific Mental Wellness Task Group, 2007, p. 8). Often repeated is the description of Inuit as a typically resilient people.

Inuit have survived for many years in one of the most challenging environments in the world, guided by a core group of values and beliefs which taught coping, endurance, connection and survival. (Korhonen, 2006, p. 4)

An Inuit healer described 'the courage, fortitude and tenacity of Inuit, of how struggle and adaptability is as much a part of the culture as legends, caribou hunting and seal skin tents' (Pauktuutit Inuit Women of Canada, 2004, p. 10). Historical and cultural pride in Inuit resilience is used as inspiration to deal with modern challenges:

We have realized that we can't keep all or our traditional culture, nor can we push away what the modern culture has given us. We must find ways to blend both to ensure that Inuit still have a future. Many of our 'tools' for survival in the social field are less practical than what you would see for survival 'tools' for going out hunting. We must determine what these tools are and integrate them with more modern ways of dealing with social issues. (Inungni Sapujjijiit Task Force on Suicide Prevention and Community Healing, 2003, p. 13)

Inuit concepts of resilience are forward-looking and stress working together. The National Strategy on Inuit Education (ITK, 2011, p. 72) outlines traditional laws for becoming 'an *inummarik*, or able human being, who can act with wisdom and use ancestral knowledge, skills and attitudes to be successful in today's world':

- Inuuqatigiitsiarniq: showing respect and caring for others;
- Tunnganarniq: being welcoming, open and inclusive;
- Piliriqatigiigniq: developing collaborative relationships to work together for a common purpose;
- Avatimik Kamattiarniq: environmental stewardship;
- Pilimmaksarniq: knowledge and skills acquisition;
- Qanuqtuurunnarniq: being resourceful to solve problems;
- Aajiqatigiiniq: consensus decision-making; and
- Pijitsirniq: serving.

The need for Inuit-specific services and Inuit control of services

Non-Inuit professionals and models have not been viewed as effective for Inuit suicide prevention:

Employees from the south don't understand our culture, traditions and don't respect our ways of dealing with issues. This is also a huge factor in our communities feeling powerless to change their situations.... Most times they can't even communicate because they don't speak the same language. (Inungni Sapujjijiit Task Force on Suicide Prevention and Community Healing, 2003, p. 24)

Inuit do not want to be fed copies of other Aboriginal programmes (Inungni Sapujjijiit Task Force on Suicide Prevention and Community Healing, 2003, p. 10). 'Aboriginal' models are most often based on First Nations cultural components (e.g. Medicine Wheel, Four Directions, sweat lodges), which have no cultural resonance with Inuit.

Alianait Inuit-specific Mental Wellness Task Group (2007, p. 11) advocated for programmes that are 'designed from an Inuit specific perspective and are adequately resourced'. Pauktuutit Inuit Women of Canada (2004, p. 11) reported how Inuit healers can relate uniquely to Inuit, because they understand what Inuit have been through and can give culturally informed advice.

The academic literature concurs about the effectiveness of Inuit controlled and Inuit-specific services:

> Evidence is accumulating to show that when Aboriginal communities, including Inuit communities, design their own interventions, typically based on traditional cultural values and practices, the efficacy of these interventions is high .... Evidence also shows that while these community based interventions are in place, suicide, even in communities with very high suicide rates, can stop altogether and other positive outcomes for youth are apparent .... (Kral *et al.*, 2009, p. 302–303)

One of the short-term outcomes desired in the Alianait Mental Wellness Action Plan is 'A pool of trained Inuit in positions across the mental wellness continuum' (Alianait Inuit-specific Mental Wellness Task Group, 2007, p. 12). Although more Inuit are completing an education than ever before, Inuit as a population have less education than other Indigenous groups in Canada (Statistics Canada, 2013). Because the need is so great and the resources small, lay counsellor training that focuses on practical skills and knowledge is needed. In addition to strengthening the numbers of professional mental health workers in Nunavut, the Government of Nunavut seeks to expand the numbers of community members trained in suicide intervention, to better equip people in communities to talk to people at risk and link them with proper care (Government of Nunavut, 2011). One such initiative is the Uqaqatigiiluk! (Talk About It) Train the Trainers programme.

Involvement of elders, youth and community

There is a need to address the issue of suicide at the community level, and to involve elders and youth. Small communities have been devastated by suicides, including copycat suicides and suicide clusters.

The generation gap is a preoccupation in the literature. Unlike the aging population of the rest of Canada, the Inuit population is primarily under 25 (Statistics Canada, 2013). Inuit youth live in a cultural and socio-economic context different than those of their parents and elders. Many speak primarily English and are active on social media, whereas elders speak primarily Inuktitut and many live in more traditional contexts.

> We lost the bond with our parents, our culture, and language in only one generation ... The people we can learn from are still there, but our lives are so different from them that it is hard to link their lives and our lives together because of the gap. (Government of Nunavut, 2009, p. 9)

In traditional Inuit life, everyone made a contribution to the well-being of the family and community, including the work of survival. Both children and elders played important roles and were valued. Elder Alicee Joamie (Inuit Tuttarvingat, 2009b, 26) contrasts this with today, in which 'There's a real disconnect between the elders and the youth'.

Solutions that work for Inuit youth must be developed with the leadership of Inuit youth (NIYC, 2010). The NIYC held a National Inuit Elders and Youth Summit in 2003, 2005, 2007 and 2010 in various parts of the Inuit Nunangat in which priorities such as language, culture, mental health, education and housing were discussed. Building local capacity to support positive lifestyles, metal wellness and to help people experiencing suicidal thoughts is particularly important in small communities, when the alternative is to send suicidal individuals out of the community or out of the territory for treatment, where the individuals are separated from family, friends, community and culture and do not necessarily heal (Inungni Sapujjijiit Task Force on Suicide Prevention and Community Healing, 2003, p. 25).

Speaking out / sharing feelings

'Speaking Out' was the first theme of eight that emerged from Inuit community consultations in Nunavut undertaken by the Inungni Sapujjijiit Task Force on Suicide Prevention and Community Healing (2003). One of the difficulties in speaking out is that in the context of intergenerational trauma and colonization, there is so much to say that has remained buried. Siasi Irqumia, Manager of the Nunalituqait Ikajuqatigiitut programme, stated:

> 'We feel a loss when we go through trauma, like death', she said, discussing her own experience with sexual abuse. 'Many people commit suicide because of unresolved trauma'.
>
> She discussed the effects of trauma at various ages and of multi-generational trauma when it is unresolved: 'Future generations become the carriers of all the unresolved trauma of the past. It becomes multiplied'. (TI, 2007, p. 9)

Unresolved anger plays a role in addictions, violence and suicide, and has cost the lives of many Inuit (TI, 2007, p. 10). Because much of the process of colonization and residential schools has remained unspoken:

> Many, many times Indigenous youth sense things are not right, but they don't know why the way things are the way they are. They have no idea what has gone on with their family members. (Weber, 2012)

A manual developed by Pauktuutit Inuit Women of Canada (2007) for Inuit shelter workers contains a segment on teaching children in shelters to name their feelings, as many have no words for what they feel and are unable to recognize the physical indications of particular emotions (tensing up, etc.). Pauktuutit Inuit Women of Canada (2007, p. 28) stated that children who grow up in violent situations must often repress their feelings, or do not know whom to trust to express their feelings.

Parenting and relationship skills

The residential school experience harmed parents in various ways. By separating them from their own parents and being taught to disrespect their parents and Inuit culture, both self-esteem and the ability to parent were lost. As well, parents' own often negative experience of schooling may continue to affect support of their own children's schooling (ITK, 2011, p. 4), which then contributes to a cycle of poverty. The following was a stark finding of the Inungni Sapujjijiit Task Force on Suicide Prevention and Community Healing (2003, p. 6):

> Our children are being raised in environments without parents because they are out gambling or out drinking all night. Our children are only showing symptoms of generations of pain and dysfunction and of how this needs to be stopped .... All too often our youth tend to feel alone.

To be clear, there are many Inuit parents who do not drink, gamble nor leave their children alone. There is also a recognition that healthy communities are needed for healthy parenting. Inuit culture includes a community role in parenting (Inungni Sapujjijiit Task Force on Suicide Prevention and Community Healing, 2003, p. 3).

The need to learn positive relationship skills and life skills in general was also frequently expressed. Inungni Sapujjijiit Task Force on Suicide Prevention and Community Healing (2003, p. 11) recommended:

> The meaning and value of healthy relationships (with oneself, with friends, between men and women, with the world) and our ability to overcome troubles – these need to be reinforced right from the start, with home supports, preschool programs, school curriculum, and child and youth opportunities for joyful experiences.

Projects adapted to Inuit priorities and realities

The results yielded many innovative suicide prevention programmes and projects that could form a separate article. On the land traditional skills programmes were viewed as particularly effective and needed (Government of Nunavut, 2011). Land-based suicide prevention programmes, where Inuit are taken out onto the tundra to learn traditional skills, provide a space to speak, listen and be heard. The *Qanuqtuurniq – Finding the Balance* interactive health promotion TV series linked Inuit live over 4.3 million square kilometers and across five time zones (Carry *et al.*, 2011, p. 4). There were circus projects, video projects and a hip hop programme (Blueprint for Life, 2013) which succeeded where other wellness outreach efforts had failed. The latter brought elders in to try their hand (or feet) at hip hop and turntable scratching, which got youth interested in listening to elders and incorporating traditional Inuit drum dancing and throat-singing into hip hop.

One of the greatest challenges facing Inuit suicide prevention is the sheer magnitude of the problem coupled with insufficient resources. For example, the Kamatsiaqtut Help Line (n.d.) which serves Nunavut and Nunavik (northern Quebec) is only staffed by volunteers for five hours per day. All the volunteers speak English, but not all speak Inuktitut or French. Urban areas where Inuit live, such as Ottawa, Montreal and Edmonton, have 24-hour crisis lines, but volunteers do not necessarily have any training in Inuit cultural contexts and the continuing effects of colonialization.

In 2012, there were sweeping funding cuts by the Canadian government to Indigenous health organizations, as a result of which the NAHO (including its Inuit specific centre, Inuit Tuttarvingat) was dismantled. Another problem is the time-limited nature of a lot of government funding. For example, the National Aboriginal Youth Suicide Prevention Strategy provided only limited project funding (Chouinard *et al.*, 2010). Many Inuit-controlled projects and services must keep reapplying for different pots of funding to try to keep operating, and sometimes have to shut down for weeks or months for lack of funds (Inuit Tuttarvingat, 2009b).

Conclusion

Whereas the general suicide prevention literature tends to examine individual risk factors such as depression, focus on intervention by professionals and suggest a range of treatment options such as pharmaceutical intervention and cognitive-behavioural therapy, the Inuit literature looks at suicide as a symptom of larger socio-economic and cultural systems, discusses suicide in the context of trauma stemming from colonialization and does not mention any role for pharmaceutical intervention, although it does not specifically oppose it. Although mental health counselling is highly valued and expressed as a need in the Inuit suicide prevention literature, the Inuit approach is based primarily on community engagement, creating cultural, socio-economic and mental wellness, emphasizing the person's strengths in the face of hardship, and putting in place programming that seeks to give youth positive experiences of life.

Colonialization had a deeply personal impact on children, parents and elders, disrupting basic family and community bonds, introducing substances such as alcohol and illicit drugs, imposing widespread trauma in terms of the physical and sexual abuse in residential schools and replacing economic, justice, religious and governance systems. It is not just the racism, it is the embodiment and internalization of the racism (Czyzewski, 2011). So the idea of 'colonial stress' as an explanation of Inuit suicide (O'Neil, 1986; Tester & McNicoll, 2004), referring to the stress of the colonized in functioning a world defined by the colonizer, with different values, cultures and languages, is a factor.

However, colonization is not just a cultural matter, but also an economic one. Europeans set up the fur trade economy in Canada, which Inuit continue to participate in, then through the activities of animal rights movements declared that the fur trade is immoral which has had a serious economic impact on Inuit (ITK, 2015). International whalers depleted the stock so that Inuit are limited in whale harvesting which was a main source of food (ITK, 2015). Climate change has affected access to other traditional foods (Statham, 2015). For many Inuit families, accessing any kind of food is difficult. The 2007–2008 International Polar Year Inuit Health Survey found that Nunavut had the highest documented rate of food insecurity – lack of regular access to food – for any Indigenous population living in a developed country in the world (Council of Canadian Academies, 2014). Widespread poverty and overcrowded housing among Inuit directly affects physical and mental health. Riva *et al.* (2014) found that overcrowded housing among Inuit led to chronic stress, sense of loss of control, which is associated with anxiety and depression. Only 42% of Inuit aged 18 to 44 have a high school diploma, compared to 89% of the Canadian population (Statistics Canada, 2013). The quality of education is also so poor that Inuit who graduate from northern high schools have difficulty continuing with their education (Bloy, 2008). As a result, many Inuit are not in a good position to integrate into the modern economy, leading to high unemployment (Statistics Canada, 2013).

The epidemic of suicide among Inuit cannot be viewed as an individual psychological matter, but as an outcome of ongoing colonization and marginalization. Loss of control, loss of culture and language, socio-economic marginalization and practices of colonization that separated families and systematically abused children are viewed as the root of suicide, violence, addictions and despair. Solutions include individual culturally sensitive mental health interventions, but as a part of a larger effort of community healing and engagement, cultural revitalization and building inclusive socio-economic structures conducive to well-being.

The work of Inuit on suicide prevention is a continually unfolding process, and the determination is unmistakable:

> We also know this from our strength as a people: *suicide is not a predetermined part of our makeup as Inuit*. The Nunavut Suicide Prevention Strategy put it very well: 'Inuit are not predisposed by virtue of ethnicity to be at a higher risk of suicide than non-Inuit'. We were not a high suicide-rate society in the past. We do not have to be a high suicide-rate society in the future. *It doesn't have to be this way.* (Audla, 2013)

Efforts by Inuit to regain control of their political, economic, educational and belief systems may contribute to suicide prevention. Efforts of Inuit to address the legacies of colonialization in terms of physical and sexual abuse; stigma, shame and internalized racism; and loss of parenting skills may contribute to suicide prevention. The magnitude of suicide among Inuit cannot simply be addressed by small-scale, time-limited programming. Systemic changes are needed. Inuit are working daily to make these systemic changes happen, but require the necessary resources to do so.

Inuit have made an enormous contribution to understanding suicide in the context of colonialization. This article is an attempt to bring some of that literature into the academic mainstream. The contribution includes the socio-economic and cultural context of suicide, the resilience model, the need to develop a positive cultural identity and the need to involve elders, youth and community in suicide prevention. A contribution of the Inuit literature to the larger suicide prevention literature is a focus not only on individual symptoms, but also on creating contexts and communities of mental wellness in which everyone has a role to play and is heard and valued.

Although this study focused on Inuit, these themes have broader implications for social work practice with clients from marginalized communities presenting with suicidal ideation. Social workers should not assume that the client is dysfunctional but that the client may be embedded in a multilevel dysfunctional situation arising from oppression of the group and how that oppression may continue to play out both in terms of socio-economic status and internalization in families and communities. Social workers can be aware that marginalized clients who come to them because of one issue may have a number of other interconnected issues to deal with. Social workers could seek out organizations associated with the client's cultural background not only for mental health resources but also for resources to increase the client's sense of pride and belonging and help with the client's socio-economic situation. Social workers can work to better link services in the community, to establish integrated services or to support any existing integrated service, such as TI in Ottawa, Canada which provides housing support, a food bank, counselling services, a medical clinic and cultural programming.

Social workers who are not from Indigenous backgrounds need to be careful about assuming what a person's cultural values are. It is also important not to suppose that all Indigenous groups share a culture, or to presume that all Indigenous clients are steeped in their traditional culture, as many may have lost touch with it. In order to help Indigenous clients, social workers can find out about Indigenous contributions to society and themselves develop a positive, but not a stereotypical, view of Indigenous cultures. Non-Indigenous social workers should never wave their knowledge or opinions about Indigenous cultures in clients' faces, or treat the client as if their ethnic background is the only important or most salient thing about them.

Learning from the Inuit focus on strengths, resilience and building positive experiences, social workers could take care to acknowledge the client's strengths and their ability to survive hardships, and that they can build on these strengths and abilities to survive to make their lives and the lives of anyone who depends on them better. A western therapeutic focus often asks the client to talk about problems or relive terrible experiences. If this approach is used, it is also very important with clients dealing with multiple challenges to facilitate positive experiences and focus on examples of where the client dealt with a challenge effectively, something the client is proud of.

Inuit are not alone in terms of Indigenous peoples who were forcibly separated from families and communities. This happened also to First Nations and Métis in Canada, to Native Americans and Alaska Natives in the USA and to Indigenous Australians. Indigenous clients affected by intergenerational trauma may benefit from skills building in healthy relationships, communication and coping strategies. Also know that the way a client may present to someone in authority, like a social worker, may be very different from how they live out other parts of their lives.

Although many social workers are trained in structural social work, it may be easy to lose touch with this approach in the daily demands of helping clients with immediate needs. The Inuit approach to suicide prevention reminds us that we need to look at community or collective approaches to healing and dealing with internalized oppression rather than just individual counselling. Suicide prevention goes beyond one-time crisis intervention, it also involves laying a strong foundation for mental and socio-economic wellness over time.

Disclosure statement

No potential conflict of interest was reported by the authors.

Note

1.   Inuk is the singular form of Inuit.

References

Alianait Inuit-specific Mental Wellness Task Group (2007) *Alianait Inuit Mental Wellness Action Plan*, Inuit Tapiriit Kanatami, Ottawa.

Audla, T. (2013) 'World suicide prevention day', 10 September 2013, Inuit Tapiriit Kanatami, Ottawa, Canada. Available at https://www.itk.ca/media (accessed 17 September 2013).

Bloy, K. (2008) 'Winnipeg Urban Inuit study, 2008', Social Planning Council of Winnipeg, Winnipeg, Canada. Available at http://www.manitobainuit.ca/pdf/Website%20-%20for%20resources%20winnipeg%20urban%20inuit%20study%202008.pdf (accessed 16 September 2014).

Blueprint for Life (2013) 'Support', Blueprint for Life, NAHO Honouring Life Network, Ilisaqsivik Society, Clyde River, Nunavut, Canada.

Carry, C. L., Clarida, K., Rideout, D., Kinnon, D. & Johnson, R. M. (2011) 'Qanuqtuurniq – finding the balance: an IPY television series using community engagement', *Polar Research*, vol. 30, no. , pp. 1–10. doi:10.3402/polar.v30i0.11514.

Chouinard, J. A., Moreau, K., Parris, S. & Cousins, J. B. (2010) 'Special study of the National Aboriginal Youth Suicide Prevention Strategy', Centre for Research on Educational and Community Services, University of Ottawa, Ottawa, Canada.

Council of Canadian Academies (2014) 'Aboriginal food security in Northern Canada: an assessment of the state of knowledge', The Expert Panel on the State of Knowledge of Food Security in Northern Canada, Council of Canadian Academies, Ottawa, Canada. Available at http://www.scienceadvice.ca/uploads/eng/assessments%20and%20publications%20and%20news%20releases/food%20security/foodsecurity_fullreporten.pdf (accessed 15 February 2015).

Czyzewski, K. (2011) Available at http://ir.lib.uwo.ca/iipj/vol2/iss1/5 (accessed 5 October 2012) 'Colonialism as a broader social determinant of health', *International Indigenous Policy Journal*, vol. 2, no. 1.

Galloway, T. & Saudny, H. (2012) *Inuit Health Survey 2007–2008 Nunavut Community and Personal Wellness*, Centre for Indigenous Peoples' Nutrition and Environment, McGill University, Montreal.

Government of Nunavut (2009) *Towards the Development of a Nunavut Suicide Prevention Strategy: A Summary Report of the 2009 Community Consultations*, Government of Nunavut, Iqaluit.

Government of Nunavut (2010) *Nunavut Suicide Prevention Strategy*, Government of Nunavut, Iqaluit.

Government of Nunavut (2011) *Nunavut Suicide Prevention Strategy Action Plan*, Government of Nunavut, Iqaluit.

Hamilton, S. M. & Rolf, K. A. (2010) 'Suicide in adolescent American Indians: preventative social work programs', *Child & Adolescent Social Work Journal*, vol. 27, no. 4, pp. 283–290. doi:10.1007/s10560-010-0204-y.

Harper, S. (2008) 'Prime Minister Harper offers full apology on behalf of Canadians for the Indian Residential Schools system', Aboriginal Affairs and Northern Development

Canada, Ottawa, Canada. Available at http://www.aadnc-aandc.gc.ca/eng/1100100015644/1100100015649 (accessed 14 September 2013).

Health Canada (2006) 'Suicide prevention', Available at http://www.hc-sc.gc.ca/fniah-spnia/promotion/suicide/index-eng.php (accessed 20 September 2013).

Hicks, J. (2007) 'The social determinants of elevated rates of suicide among Inuit youth', *Indigenous Affairs*, vol. 4, pp. 30–37.

Inuit Tuttarvingat (2009a) 'How are we as men?', *Qanuqtuurniq – Finding the Balance* television series and DVD, Iqaluit, Nunavut, Inuit Communications (ICSL), Canada. Available at http://www.naho.ca/wellnessTV/documents/InuitMenTVTranscript.pdf (accessed 5 September 2013).

Inuit Tuttarvingat (2009b) 'I am young and I am proud', *Qanuqtuurniq – Finding the Balance* television series and DVD, Iqaluit, Nunavut, Inuit Communications (ICSL), Canada. Available at http://www.naho.ca/wellnessTV/documents/2010-10-19_YouthTVShowDVDTranscript-Final.pdf (accessed 6 September 2013).

Inungni Sapujjijiit Task Force on Suicide Prevention and Community Healing (2003) 'Our words must come back to us', Nunavut Department of Health and Social Services, Iqaluit, Nunavut, Canada.

ITK (Inuit Tapiriit Kanatami) (2011) *First Canadians, Canadians First: National Strategy on Inuit Education 2011*, Inuit Tapiriit Kanatami, Ottawa.

ITK (2015) 'Inuit and Europeans', Available at https://www.itk.ca/about-inuit/inuit-and-europeans (accessed 15 February 2015).

Jacobson, J. M., Osteen, P. J., Sharpe, T. L. & Pastoor, J. B. (2012) 'Randomized trial of suicide gatekeeper training for social work students', *Research on Social Work Practice*, vol. 22, no. 3, pp. 270–281. doi:10.1177/1049731511436015.

Jokinen, J., Forslund, K., Ahnemark, E., Gustavsson, J. P., Nordström, P. & Åsberg, M. (2010) 'Karolinska Interpersonal Violence Scale predicts suicide in suicide attempters', *Journal of Clinical Psychiatry*, vol. 71, no. 8, pp. 1025–1032. doi:10.4088/JCP.09m05944blu.

Kamatsiaqtut Help Line (n.d.) 'Kamatsiaqtut', Available at http://www.nnsl.com/nunavutnews/Kamatsiaqtut.pdf (accessed 9 September 2013).

Kirmayer, L. J., Fletcher, C. & Boothroyd, L. J. (1998) 'Suicide among the Inuit of Canada', in *Suicide in Canada*, eds A. A. Leenaars, S. Wenkstern, I. Sakinofsky, R. J. Dyck, M. J. Kral & R. C. Bland, University of Toronto Press, Toronto, pp. 187–211.

Korhonen, M. (2006) *Suicide Prevention: Inuit Traditional Practices that Encouraged Resilience and Coping*, Ajunnginiq Centre/Inuit Tuttarvingat of the National Aboriginal Health Organization, Ottawa.

Korhonen, M. (2007) *Resilience: Overcoming Challenges and Moving on Positively*, Ajunnginiq Centre/Inuit Tuttarvingat, National Aboriginal Health Organization, Ottawa.

Kral, M. J., Wiebe, P. K., Nisbet, K., Dallas, C., Okalik, L., Enuaraq, N. & Cinotta, J. (2009) 'Canadian Inuit community engagement in suicide prevention', *International Journal of Circumpolar Health*, vol. 68, no. 3, pp. 292–308. doi:10.3402/ijch.v68i3.18330.

NIYC (National Inuit Youth Council) (2010) 'Inuit youth embrace life on world suicide prevention day', Available at http://www.niyc.ca/news/inuit-youth-embrace-life-world-suicide-prevention-day (accessed 12 September 2013).

NIYC (2012) 'NIYCs 6th Annual Inuit celebration of life', Available at http://www.niyc.ca/news/niycs-6th-annual-inuit-celebration-life (accessed 12 September 2013).

Oliver, L. N., Peters, P. A. & Kohen, D. E. (2012) 'Mortality rates among children and teenagers living in Inuit Nunangat, 1994 to 2008', *Health Reports*, 18 July 2012. Available at http://www.statcan.gc.ca/pub/82-003-x/2012003/article/11695-eng.pdf (accessed 1 October 2012).

O'Neil, J. (1986) 'Colonial stress in the Canadian Arctic: an ethnography of young adults changing', in *Anthropology and Epidemiology*, eds C. R. Janes, R. Stall & S. M. Giford, Reidel Publishing, Dordrecht/Boston, MA/Lancaster/Tokyo.

Osteen, P. J., Jacobson, J. M. & Sharpe, T. L. (2014) 'Suicide prevention in social work education: how prepared are social work students?', *Journal of Social Work Education*, vol. 50, no. 2, pp. 349–364.

Pauktuutit Inuit Women of Canada (2004) 'Inuit healing in contemporary Inuit society', Pauktuutit Inuit Women of Canada, Ottawa, Canada. Available at http://pauktuutit.ca/wp-content/blogs.dir/1/assets/AHFNuluaqInuitHealing_e.pdf (accessed 4 February 2013).

Pauktuutit Inuit Women of Canada (2007) *Making Our Shelters Strong: Training for Inuit Shelter Workers Participant Handbook*, Pauktuutit Inuit Women of Canada, Ottawa.

PHAC (Public Health Agency of Canada) (2012) 'The Chief Public Health Officer's report on the State of Public Health in Canada, 2011', Public Health Agency of Canada, Ottawa, Canada. Available at http://www.phac-aspc.gc.ca/cphorsphc-respcacsp/2011/index-eng.php (accessed 30 September 2012).

Riva, M., Plusquellec, P., Juster, R.-P., Laouan-Sidi, E. A., Abdous, B., Lucas, M., Dery, S. & Dewailly, E. (2014) 'Household crowding is associated with higher allostatic load among the Inuit', *Journal of Epidemiology & Community Health*, 2 January. Available at http://jech.bmj.com/content/early/2014/01/02/jech-2013-203270 (accessed 15 February 2015)/doi:10.1136/jech-2013-203270.

Royal Commission on Aboriginal Peoples (1996) *Report of the Royal Commission on Aboriginal Peoples*, Government of Canada, Ottawa.

Ruth, B. J., Gianino, M., Muroff, J., McLaughlin, D. & Feldman, B. N. (2012) 'You can't recover from suicide: perspectives on suicide education in MSW programs', *Journal of Social Work Education*, vol. 48, no. 3, pp. 501–516. doi:10.5175/JSWE.2012.201000095.

Scott, M. (2015) 'Teaching note – understanding of suicide prevention, intervention, and postvention: curriculum for MSW students', *Journal of Social Work Education*, vol. 51, no. 1, pp. 177–185.

Statham, S. (2015) 'Inuit food security: vulnerability of the traditional food system to climatic extremes', Climate Change Adaptation Research Group, McGill University. Available at http://ccadapt.ca/sarafoodsecurity/ (accessed 15 February 2013).

Statistics Canada (2013) *Aboriginal Peoples in Canada: First Nations People, Métis and Inuit*, Minister of Industry, Ottawa.

Tester, F. J. & McNicoll, P. (2004) 'Isumagijaksaq: mindful of the state: social constructions of Inuit suicide', *Social Science and Medicine*, vol. 58, no. 12, pp. 2625–2636. doi:10.1016/j.socscimed.2003.09.021.

TI (Tungasuvvingat Inuit) (2007) *Mamisarniq Conference 2007 Inuit-specific Approaches to Healing from Addiction and Trauma*, Inuit Tapiriit Kanatami, Ottawa.

Weber, B. (2012) 'NWT, Nunavut to launch mandatory classes on residential schools', *The Globe and Mail*, 3 October. Available at http://www.theglobeandmail.com/news/national/education/nwt-nunavut-to-launch-mandatory-classes-on-residential-schools/article4587588/ (accessed 30 October 2012).

Wexler, L., Gubrium, A., Griffin, M. & DiFulvio, G. (2013) 'Promoting positive youth development and highlighting reasons for living in Northwest Alaska through digital storytelling', *Health Promotion Practice*, vol. 14, no. 4, pp. 617–623. doi:10.1177/1524839912462390.

Martin Stuart Smith

'ONLY CONNECT' 'NEAREST RELATIVE'S' EXPERIENCES OF MENTAL HEALTH ACT ASSESSMENTS

This article begins with a description of the role of the 'nearest relative' in relation to people who are assessed under the Mental Health Act 1983. The rights conferred by this role are defined and explained, and some contentious aspects of the role are highlighted. A discussion about customer satisfaction responses to services provided then follows, both generally and specifically in the context of Health and Social Care. Examples are given of feedback from relatives of people who have encountered mental health crisis services and from service users themselves. A customer satisfaction survey is then described in which 32 nearest relatives gave telephone interviews about their contact with Approved Mental Health Professionals (AMHPs) using the Mental Health Act. The findings demonstrate that, while experiences of the AMHPs were generally positive, the qualities of empathy, explanation, understanding, caring and support were valued particularly highly.

The role of the 'nearest relative'

Most people assessed under the terms of The Mental Health Act 1983 (MHA) will have a 'nearest relative' as defined by section 26 of this Act. Patients cannot choose their nearest relative and, apart from in exceptional circumstances, nearest relatives cannot choose this role for themselves. When someone is assessed under the MHA their nearest relative will usually be the person at the top of the following list:

husband, wife or civil partner,
son or daughter (aged over 18),
father or mother,
brother or sister,
grandparent,
grandchild,
uncle or aunt and
nephew or niece.

If the patient 'ordinarily resides with or is cared for by' one or more of his relatives that relative/those relatives will be given preference over the other relatives on the list. If the patient has both relatives available on the list above, e.g. a father and a mother, preference is given to the elder of the two (section 26 MHA).

The nearest relative has several powers conferred by the MHA. While nearly all applications for admission under the MHA are made by an Approved Mental Health Professional (AMHP), the nearest relative can apply (section 11 MHA). However, in practice this option is exercised very rarely (Jones, 2013, p. 86). One of the reasons for this is so that the patient cannot claim at a later date that their relative has 'sectioned' them as the decision to apply is not usually made by the nearest relative but by an AMHP with a more professionally detached 'objective' view of the patient and their circumstances. The AMHP has a duty to inform the nearest relative that an application might be made or has been made (section 11 MHA) but it is the decision of the AMHP and the assessing Doctors as to whether the patient is admitted to hospital and not the nearest relatives. The AMHP's duty is to consult and not necessarily to agree with the preference the relative states. Jones (2013, p. 89) cites,

> The consultation will have two objectives. The first will be to provide information to the AMHP to assist with the decision of whether to apply for admission. The second will be to put the nearest relative in a position to object to an application.

In my experience as an AMHP nearest relatives are more likely to request that the patient be admitted to hospital and this not be agreed than to oppose admission and this be arranged. Although the rights and duties of the MHA make these roles clear the feelings of the patient might be that they have been 'sectioned' and possibly therefore betrayed by their nearest relative while the relative might continue to feel guilty in relation to a decision that was not (legally) made by them when an AMHP has made the application. The AMHP should be aware of the possibility of these powerful underlying, irrational feelings as well as the clear demarcation of responsibilities and roles identified by the MHA.

The nearest relative cannot prevent an application for a section 2 (admission for assessment, maximum 28 day order) being made although they can object to it subsequently. They can prevent an application being made for a section 3 (admission for treatment, maximum 6 month order) unless they are displaced or attempts to consult with them 'are not reasonably practicable or would involve unreasonable delay' (section 11 MHA). The nearest relative also has the right to require an AMHP to 'consider the patient's case with a view to making application for his admission to hospital' (section 13 MHA).

One of the primary reasons for AMHPs needing to contact nearest relatives is that the nearest relative is assumed to have (relatively) detailed knowledge about the patient and also to have their best interests at heart. Speaking to someone who knows how the patient usually thinks and acts, and therefore being assisted to frame the recent behaviours that have brought the patient to attention in some kind of context is valuable for AMHPs. This is particularly the case when there might be no known recorded/available history and/or when the patient is being assessed out of hours by two Doctors and an AMHP who have never met them previously. The ideal nearest relative will act as an informed advocate for the patient and those close to the patient as well as giving a compassionate view about what they think the patient needs most at the point of assessment. However, the assumption that the nearest relative will always have the patient's best interests at heart would be tested, for example, in relation to a patient who forbids the AMHP to make contact with their relative, claiming that this relative had abused them in some way (see discussion of 'R.(on the application of E) v Bristol City Council (2005') in Jones, 2013, p. 91). In these instances there is a balance to strike between the relative's right to be consulted (see above) and the patient's right to confidentiality as well as private and family life under article 8 of the Human Rights Act 1998. The case could be further complicated by the assessing AMHP and Doctors not knowing whether such claims against a relative are founded on fact or might be a manifestation of a patient's illness.

Another aspect of contact with nearest relatives I have found interesting when working as AMHP is the stipulation that if both relatives of a pair listed in section 26 MHA are available then the AMHP should consult with the elder of the two. For example, when a patient has both a father and mother available as a potential nearest relative, if the father is the elder (and has/had parental responsibility for the patient) the AMHP should speak with him. However, I have had many conversations with fathers who have said as soon as they can, 'I'll just pass you over to my wife'. I have then needed to explain that while I can talk to their wife as well as them it is only them who has the legally defined role of nearest relative. In other families a wife might be older than her husband but the husband is takes the role of making decisions regarding the family and household rather than the wife in which cases the wife wants to defer to her husband. Similarly a patient is not necessarily closest to their eldest sibling or eldest child. While there is no easy, 'one size fits all' way of defining which relative is truly (rather than legally) 'nearest' to the patient the reversion to the 'eldest' in all cases is a crude and sometimes inaccurate measure of closeness.

This discussion has highlighted the importance of the role of nearest relatives for AMHPs when undertaking assessments under the MHA and recognition of this provided an impetus to write this paper. A brief review of social work literature relevant to the nearest relative role is now considered.

Literature

A particular and detailed consideration of the role of the nearest relative is absent from much of the social work literature. The importance of the family context into which patients are discharged from hospital and the part played by the 'high expressed emotion' that might be expressed in these contexts and contribute to re-admission is well documented (for example, Leff, 2001). However, this does not amount to a discussion of the 'nearest' relative role. Tew et. al. (2012, p. 451) reviewing the evidence relating to social factors and recovery from mental health difficulties acknowledge the importance of connectedness by way of" inter-personal relationships", but again, the nearest relative, specifically, is not mentioned. This is also the case with Beecher's paper (2009) which considers the importance of 'the family' of the patient but not the nearest relative. Dwyer (2012) writes of 'walking the tightrope of a mental health act assessment' from the AMHP's perspective, but her focus is not on the part played by nearest relatives in these assessments.

The nearest relative is not mentioned in Nathan and Weber's (2010) consideration of mental health social work and the bureau-medicalisation of mental health care, Pilgrim's (2009) discussion about recovery from mental health problems or Uttarkar's (2010) investigation into the experiences of community mental health staff. Hewitt (2010a, 2010b) has written specifically of the nearest relative's role in objecting to their relative being detained under the MHA and Berzins and Atkinson (2009) have considered how the role of the 'named person' (the equivalent of the nearest relative in Scottish law) is viewed by service users and carers.

Cameron and McGowan's (2013, p. 27), 'The mental health social worker as transitional participant' is relevant to this paper in that it considers how the social worker (AMHP in this case) can function as transitional participant 'who can usefully bridge and integrate the disparate aspects of the . . . determined social (external) and subjective emotional (internal) environments of their clients'. It is bridging these two aspects of experience that the AMHP is attempting when talking with nearest relatives.

Although the nearest relative is not the focus of Gregory and Thompson's paper concerning a service user's experiences through a mental health crisis (2013, p. 460) the authors show vividly how crucial different relatives can be at a time of acute distress:

> 'I feared my partner was going to kill me, because later that day he went to stay with my ex-husband and son. My sister had to return to work, and so my father volunteered to come and stay with me to look after me. After the various professionals had left, I remember sitting outside and having lunch with my father and sister and feeling a lot calmer. Later in the evening my son visited. I remember him saying to me 'My stepdad wouldn't hurt you mummy' but at that time I was not able to believe that'

This extract also illustrates how many different relatives can be involved with a service user at any one time. It is sometimes the case that the person with the role of the 'nearest' relative is not necessarily the person who the service user is closest to or the one they would choose to represent their interests.

Gregory and Thompson's account (2013) also provides an example of the service user feedback that can count so powerfully in forming perceptions about service delivery. This increasingly influential aspect of contemporary living is now considered.

From victim to owner: keeping the customer satisfied in the worlds of Health and Social Care

Service user feedback has gained momentum as a prevailing force and influence over recent years. The *Trip Advisor* feedback recorded as service user's experience is a first port of call for many considering whether or not to use a particular service. What services have to say about themselves in their publicity is seen as less important than the comments of others who have used the service. Increasingly, the message to consumers is 'You need to know what other people say they think about this'.

I recently noticed a poster advertising a film. There was a picture of a man standing by a railway track with a rifle across his shoulders. He looked intent and unhappy. The title of the film was displayed in large letters. Other than that there was no information at all about the film but there were the names of six different publications with the number of stars (all high) they had awarded the film next to the name of the publication. AB rates this film four stars, CD, five stars, EF, four stars … I thought the message to me was that I don't need to know what the film is about right now but I do need to know what other people think of it. Having returned from seeing a film (not unduly influenced into seeing it from the comments of others I hope!) after a short time I received a text message asking me to comment on the film. Will I send in a review? Similarly, with many purchases. Will I submit a review? Here's an incentive … Driving behind a large lorry I see a message on the back of it. 'How am I driving? 'Phone xxxx'. The interests in service user feedback in contemporary culture look like they are here to stay and they are establishing a firmer hold and more persuasive influence as time goes on.

It seems to me that Health and Social care services often struggle to keep up with the demands to show 'customer satisfaction' ratings of their services to the same extent as the Private sector. To some extent this might be because people who use these services would not choose to use them at all, if given a choice. As Campbell puts it, 'Numerous recipients of crisis services are not just unwilling recipients but are compelled recipients' (Read & Reynolds, 2000, p. 180). The fact that there is this *involuntary* aspect to being forced to use services, or having services 'forced' upon them, is a significant feature here. By definition, people assessed under MHA have not asked for this to happen, as if they were thought to need hospital admission and had agreed to this they would become voluntary patients and thus avoid the need for formal assessment under the MHA. Similarly, most nearest relatives have not chosen or agreed to take this role. The role is determined for them by section 26 MHA as outlined above. Therefore the involuntary and possibly unwilling and compelled aspects of the role are inherent in it.

Service users who have a positive experience of being assessed and treated under the MHA are unlikely to want to advertise this after the event, whereas those who perceive their experiences as being poor or wanting are more likely to raise this in available forums. This results in the service user feedback that does exist being predominantly negative. Reading *The Big Issue in the North 15–21 September 2014* I noticed an advert on p. 34 which simply read, 'Have you had trouble with social workers? Telephone xxxx'. I noticed my instinctive response to this advert was to feel somewhat anxious and threatened. I mentioned this to a colleague who replied, 'Surely the advert is a good thing as it will help to bring to light bad practice'. Despite appreciating the point she was making I was also aware of a shadow side of customer feedback in that some people might use it to attack social workers who are struggling with a lack of resources, inadequate supervision and support and overwhelming work pressures. 'These people need understanding and support' I thought, 'Not, further criticism'. I was interested to note this reaction arising in myself. Although sufficiently committed to the importance of gaining service user feedback to write this article I also and simultaneously had concerns about how this feedback might be used/interpreted.

The first significant study recording service user feedback of those who used social care (family welfare) services was published as 'The Client Speaks' (Mayer & Timms, 1970). Since then there have been several other publications in increasing numbers as the 'Trip Advisor' mentality asserts itself deeper into popular culture (see Wilson *et al.*

(2011) and Ruch *et al.* (2010) for summaries of these). Writing in 2005 Tew refers to 'An almost unprecedented interest in service user perspectives. The buzz words are; "involvement", "inclusion", "empowerment" and "partnership"' (p. 32). A Concordat aimed at improving outcomes for people experiencing mental crisis has recently been published by the Department of Health (2014). This publication states there should be,

> a thematic review of the quality, safety and responsiveness of care provided to people experiencing a mental health crisis by regulated providers and provider agencies with responsibility for operating the MHA 1983 ... The desired outcome of this is that service users experience more appropriate and consistent responses, disseminating latest best practice evidence and emerging case studies. (pp. 49, 53)

Reviewing what service users have generally found positive from social work involvement Ruch *et al.* (2010, p. 199) identify the following:

*   understanding the intentions and purposes of the worker,
*   contributing to the work of the service,
*   receiving help speedily,
*   the worker's ability to respond to feelings not always expressed,
*   the worker's concern and attention, even if change is not possible and
*   the worker's ability to exercise care, even when exercising control.

Hardcastle *et al.* (2007, p. 78) show how relatives of mental health service users can feel guilt, fear, despair and anger. One father writes poignantly of his experience:

> 'The worst thing that happened in my life was having my son admitted to hospital against his will ... The hardest thing I did was to help the police put handcuffs on him. It was the only way to help him at the time, but the memory of doing that will stay with me for the rest of my life ... I 'phoned my wife. She couldn't stop crying, and I felt I needed to be there to support her, but wanted to find out what was happening. I felt really torn, feeling in need of support myself, but having so many people who needed my support ... My son had lots of odd ideas about what had been going on in the weeks before he was admitted, some of them relating to other family members ... I know we did not always come across as reasonable, but at the beginning we were in shock, and later on we couldn't understand what was happening. I would have thought they would have understood our emotions better ...' (Hardcastle, 2007, pp. 80–82).

This brief extract contains several telling points in relation to a relative's experiences of a family member's crisis. We do not know the age of the father or the son but note that the father described the experience as 'the worst thing that happened' in his life. One does not get to be a father without collecting several distressing life experiences but this was the worst. He claims the (bad) memories of his involvement will stay with him for the rest of his life. However much he could rationalise that he did the 'right' thing for his son at the time, the feeling he is left with is a deep sense of his actions being fundamentally 'wrong'. Those he would usually look to for support (for example, his wife) need him to support them. He feels 'torn' – a word that has visceral resonance when used in this context. The father expresses an aspect of wondering how others might see him and other family members because of the 'odd ideas' his son had been giving voice to. He knows he was not 'reasonable' but felt as if his capacity for reason had deserted him and been supplanted by a feeling of (chaotic) shock. He therefore looks for understanding from those dealing with him but does not find it.

A mother writes of suddenly finding herself lonely and abandoned in a world she did not choose and does not want to inhabit,

> 'In this new situation of a mental health problem, I had neither love nor support, and did not know where to find help. There was no one with whom I could share this burden. The whole territory of mental health problems was strange, unpredictable and frightening; my world had become as surreal as my daughter's … My daughter was upset and very angry that I had caused her to be sectioned; she and I were both in tears, I recall a nurse standing by irritated and impatient that we were not just getting on with it … ' (Hardcastle *et al.* 2007, pp. 95, 96).

As with the father cited above, this mother finds herself unsupported and not knowing where to go to for help. She feels cut off; *torn* from possibilities of support, 'There was *no one* with whom I could share this'. As well as the hurt and pain, this mother experiences a surreal aspect to what is happening to her. This reads like the kind of denial that often accompanies trauma, 'This *can't* be happening … '. There is another sense in which she identifies with and is implicated in what was happening to her daughter. She refers to the guilt and the blame that many relatives feel that they have 'caused' their relative to be sectioned, even though in most cases legally, it is not their decision or their signature on the application form. The comment about the nurse's irritation and impatience echoes that of the father quoted above; 'I would have thought they would have understood our emotions better'. A difficulty faced by those in the caring professions is that mental health assessments and admissions are a bureaucratic-administrative process as well as an emotional experience and there is frequently a tension when attempting to address all aspects of this process at the same time. This is why the qualities of workers showing concern and attention, even if change is not possible along with an ability to exercise care, even when exercising control cited by Ruch *et al.* (2010) above are valued by service users.

Reflecting on the experience of the father cited above a psychologist comments,

> 'Why is it that the staff described seem unempathic, unable to put themselves in the other's shoes, to tune into emotion, or to act in a way that is not defensive?. Mental health staff should bring a calmness, a reassuring presence, should be the holders of hope for those in distress' (Hardcastle *et.al.* 2007, p. 86).

In what ways and to what extent reassurance and hope are ultimately or actually valuable is debatable (Smith, 2000) but the point is well made that the father (and the mother) quoted above did not seem to receive the support or understanding they felt in need of from others at the time.

The extent to which relatives of those who come attention to the Mental Health Services can feel disorientated, lost and alone is considerable. This is conveyed by a mother who uses a powerful metaphor when talking of her experiences with her son's mental illness, 'You learn to cope, that's all you do. *You're living on the edge of the world sometimes* ... ' (Heller *et al.* 1996, p. 100). The patient's sister articulates what she and her mother would have liked from professionals, 'You need somebody who will sit down, and you can say, 'How can we deal with this, how are we meant to react, what do you want us to do? ... ' (Heller *et al.* 1996, p. 98). The 'somebody who will sit down' is a different person to the nurse described above as being irritated and impatient. It will not be possible for professionals to answer the questions, 'How should we react? What should we do?' but the desire of the relatives to have someone available to them, to 'sit with' them while they attempt to digest and make sense of what is happening is apparent. The edge of the world sounds like a frightening place to be ...

In a chapter entitled, 'What we want from crisis services' Read and Reynolds (2000, p. 181) cite a service user who claims:

- People want more control, particularly more of their own control over crisis situations.
- People want to gain understanding of and from their crises.
- People want to be treated with respect and dignity.

Or, in the words of another service user, quoted by Laurence (2003, p. 137), 'you [want to] stop being a victim of your experience and start being the owner of your experience'

Motivated, partly by the anticipated value of researching nearest relative's views of their experiences of mental health crises and partly by wanting to see if there were any improvements that could be made to AMHP practice in a County in Southern England a customer satisfaction survey was devised and carried out. This survey and its findings are now described.

Methodology, sample, questions asked, analysis of data

Attempts were made to contact 42 nearest relatives of people assessed under MHA 1983 out of normal office hours in a County in Southern England in between July and September 2014. Nearest relatives were asked to participate in a telephone interview conducted by an experienced administrative worker, independent of the team for which the AMHPs worked, but knowledgeable about the workings of the team.

A qualitative methodology using telephone interviews was chosen. This was because I was interested in ascertaining from the relatives, how they *experienced* their contacts with the AMHPs, and given them opportunity to talk about their thoughts and feelings in their own words. I knew from experience that previous attempts to obtain service user's views by sending them a list of questions and asking them to respond resulted in a poor response rate and that a qualitative methodology would serve my purpose best (Smith, 2000). I also knew from my contact with nearest relatives that most would respond well to a telephone call, even one they were not expecting, and be able to talk pertinently, and in detail, about their relative. In this respect the methodology and method of the research followed social work practice.

Ethical problems were not anticipated and did not arise as people contacted were known to the service and were free to decline to take part in the research. In fact, several relatives said they were pleased to have been contacted and given the opportunity to give their views and talk further about their experiences. The administrative worker and I kept in close contact throughout the research so that she could raise any problems/ethical issues arising with me if there were any. An advantage of the administrative worker contacting the relatives rather than me was that it introduced an independence and objectivity into the process so that I was not seen as 'checking up on' AMHPs who I managed. Data obtained was analysed by way of inductive thematic analysis and seeing what themes of importance emerged from the questions asked (Whittaker, 2009).

Of the 42 relatives contacted, ten relatives either did not respond to attempts to contact them or said they did not want to participate in the survey. Thirty two relatives were therefore interviewed.

The administrator read the following script before each interview,

'Hello, I'm xx from xy County Council. Would you have a few minutes to answer some questions about your recent involvement with the Out of Hours Emergency Social Work team, (name amhp) who spoke to you about your relative (name) on (date)'

She then asked participants who agreed to be interviewed the following questions:

1. How clear did you find the duty social worker was when speaking to you and providing information?
2. Were they polite?
3. Did they give you all the information you wanted/needed throughout the process of your relative being assessed?
4. Were there aspects of the worker's communication that you thought were particularly good or bad?
5. Could their communication with you have been improved in any way?
6. Do you have any further comments that could help us to improve our out of hours service to members of the public?

These questions were chosen as they asked about aspects of experience most important to service users and also provided them with an opportunity to make suggestions about how the contact with them and the AMHP service generally could be improved.

Responses to questions

1. Not very clear: 2, Fairly clear: 4, Clear: 9, Very clear: 17.
2. Polite: 24, Very polite: 8.
3. Yes, provided full information: 26. No, did not provide full information: 4. N/A: 2.
4. Comments made about good/bad communication:

Positive comments about the AMHPs communication referred to their patience, willingness to discuss information/issues, calmness, good level of understanding, good 'bedside manner, supportiveness, calmness and re-assurance at a stressful time. Empathy, clarity, keeping relatives 'in the loop', openness/approachability and waiting with relatives were also mentioned.

Aspects of communication found to be not so helpful were that the AMHP's accent was difficult to follow/understand, and, at times AMHPs were experienced as vague and evasive (this was acknowledged by relatives as possibly being due to the AMHP's need to maintain confidentiality). Not being informed of the outcome of an assessment and the desire for more detailed information/feedback were also mentioned.

5. Suggestions for improved communication.

In response to this question relatives indicated that there was a need to be aware that they might be tired and distressed and therefore not able to 'hear' what was being said to them, even if and when this was communicated clearly. Relatives also mentioned that they would have liked more information about how to access support for themselves and clearer instructions about how to locate the hospital.

6. Comments to help improve the service provided by the Out of Hours AMHPs.

Relatives referred to the need for a proportionate and efficient response from call handlers taking telephone calls before they got through to speak to an AMHP directly. The difficulty of talking about sensitive issues, particularly with the patient present was mentioned as is indicated in the following response, 'I felt unsafe about the questions asked about my children. I was not happy overall about how my partner had been treated. It was difficult to talk about some things with my partner present'.

Several relatives commented that they felt services had generally 'gone downhill', been cut back or were less available than they had been in previous years. Because of this there is a particular need for AMHPs to oversee and communicate an effective handover to a responsive day time follow-up service. Long waits that fuelled anxieties were also mentioned with relatives citing waits of 12 and 14 hours before the patient was assessed.

Some situations changed quickly, leaving relatives having to adapt to different requests/expectations,

'We were contacted around 3 am, initially my relative was assessed as being fit enough to be discharged to the care of my husband and myself. We are both senior citizens and were not happy about this due to previous experience but agreed to attend the police station to collect our relative. We received another phone call before we had finished getting dressed to inform us the situation had escalated and our relative was being admitted to hospital'.

Some relatives found the exclusivity of the nearest relative role frustrating, 'After the assessment another social worker contacted us for an update but would not speak with my husband because I am legally the Nearest Relative, it was upsetting at such a difficult time'. This is particularly likely to be the case when 'nearest' does not necessarily mean 'dearest' and when the person who happens to the nearest relative is not necessarily the most available/ interested/involved in their relative's care.

Several relatives expressed appreciation of the AMHP service as it was provided to them. Bearing in mind the negative portrayals of social workers in much media coverage, several relatives interviewed for this survey reported positive experiences of their contact with the AMHP service:

'The AMHP was very good, just brilliant – I couldn't fault them in any way'

'AMHP was great, good as they could be in the circumstances'

'They were there, I don't know what I would have done without them. They were so helpful – fantastic'.

'AMHP was very clear and helpful'

Some relatives expressed pleasure at being able to give positive feedback about their experience and these responses provided a justification for and validation of the telephone interviews conducted. An example of this type of response is:

'Given the situation AMHP did very well, and handled a demanding task well.

As a carer I would like to say I don't know how the system works, there have been changes and there should be more information about new arrangements. I am very pleased to have been called and would be pleased to be contacted again'.

Analysis

After the completion of the survey I spoke with the administrative worker who had asked the questions what general impressions she had formed about the contact that the AMHPs had with the nearest relatives and what impressions she had gained about the strengths and weaknesses of the service offered. She told me that the response of the relatives was generally positive. She had found most relatives were willing, even keen, to talk to her about their experiences of their relative being assessed. Even if the assessment was some time ago the memories of the process of assessment remained vividly with many relatives. After speaking with the administrator I found the following account from a relative recorded in Hardcastle *et al.* (2007, p. 105)

We had a phone call around 10.30 pm to report an incident which took months off our recovery. Even now, phone calls after 10.00 pm send a feeling of dread through our systems – the chest still tightens, things are, even now, only just under the surface.

The words 'even now' are repeated in a short space of time in this extract and it is this 'ongoingness' of an experience which has ostensibly passed, 'just under the surface' that the administrator had picked up.

For people who had encountered the mental health services for the first time there was a sense of them having been considerably shaken up and disturbed by the experience (the worker said, 'Not traumatised, exactly...' twice when describing these responses). Because of this the relatives seemed to value the 'empathising, explaining, understanding, caring and supporting' they experienced from the AMHPs. Specifically, they valued a calming response that 'helped them not to panic too much', outlined what was happening at the point of contact and what would happen next. The most commonly reported issue for relatives was when they couldn't readily understand the accent of the AMHP who was speaking to them, particularly as such sensitive matters were being discussed.

Some relatives said that they thought the quantity, quality and 'clarity' of ongoing support services had 'gone downhill' recently. They said they were aware of lots of changes taking place very quickly to the extent that they no longer knew who to ask for support or where to go in order to access this support.

Implications for practice

The AMHPS working for this particular out of hours team were skilled and experienced workers and their sensitivity and skills in communication are apparent from several of the comments listed above. In terms of improving the service yet further, there are the following implications for practice:

- AMHPS should be mindful of their accents and how these might not be readily understood particularly when conveying complex information in a short time.
- AMHPs should remember that relatives might be tired, stressed and distracted so take care and time to convey information briefly and clearly.
- The relative's need for support, assistance and guidance in their own right should be considered.
- As much information/feedback as possible should be provided, within the context of data protection, along with recognition that relatives might not take it all in the first time of being told.
- AMHPs should offer relatives a telephone number they can contact for further ongoing discussion/information even if this is not the AMHP's own number.
- Although the provision of longer-term responses are not the responsibility or remit of the AMHP they should be aware of the state of confusion about support services experienced by several relatives currently and advise/ guide them through options as clearly as possible.

Conclusion: 'Only connect'

This article has illustrated the need to take the views and perspectives of nearest relatives into account when carrying out assessments under The MHA. The Care Act 2014 places further requirements on Local Authorities to consider and address the needs of carers (and therefore nearest relatives) and so these aspects of social work will be important to develop over the coming years in areas wider than mental health services.

A theme emerging consistently from the literature cited about the experiences of nearest relatives and service users is the importance of the relationship that is established with the AMHP and other professionals. Even when a relationship is not ongoing, a relatively brief one-off interaction can contribute significantly to the enduring memories of the relatives involved. Much has been written about the value of relationship based social work practice recently (see Ruch *et al.* (2010), Wilson *et al.* (2011) and these more recent writings echo formative texts underpinning the values of social work and casework from the profession's earlier days. Biestek (1967, p. 106) writes,

'[Ideally] the caseworker opens doors and windows to let in air, light and sunshine, so that the client can breathe more easily and see more clearly. The aim is to help him gain a better insight into his problem, and develop strength to help himself'.

Air, light and sunshine might be hard to find at the dark and difficult times that characterise many MHA assessments but the objective of helping nearest relatives 'breathe more easily and see more clearly' so that they can assume more mastery and control about the combination of circumstances they face should be valued.

While trends and fashions in social work and mental health thinking come and go, the essential needs of people in crisis have changed relatively little since earliest civilizations. Biestek (1967, p. 135) claims, 'All human beings have certain common basic needs: physical, emotional, intellectual, social and spiritual. In adverse circumstances these common needs are felt with a special poignancy.' It is at times of these adverse circumstances when needs are felt with a special poignancy by both mental health service users and their nearest relatives that the qualities of empathy, explanation, understanding, caring and support identified above are particularly valued. In the words of a service user, quoted in Read and Reynolds 2000, p. 183, 'In my view, the crucial questions about mental health crisis services are to do not with locations and technology but with understandings'.

One of the reasons why these understandings are so vital is that service users and their relatives often feel profoundly isolated when touched by mental illness. The metaphor of the prison which cuts people off from sustaining contact with others pervades descriptions of what it feels like to be in a world where mental illness features (Rowe, 2003). Understandings create connections which help people feel less alone and cut off. It is sometimes difficult for AMHPs and other professional workers to communicate understandings and connections when they are trying to manage and balance the details of a legal process, the perceived illness of the service user, the (sometimes extremely strong) feelings and emotions of nearest relatives and their own personal resonances to experiences. The personal experiences of the worker might only be partly understood by the worker themselves so that they experience their counter-transference reactions to patents, their relatives and their situations as confusing and disorientating (Winnicott, 1947/1987; Colman, 1989, Obholzer & Roberts, 1997). Establishing connections with service users and their relatives does not resolve these complex and multifaceted difficulties but it does help people feel less alone when confronted with them. At least this constitutes a place to start from …

Acknowledgements

With thanks to Marilyn Anderson who conducted the telephone interviews reported in this article.

Disclosure statement

No potential conflict of interest was reported by the author.

References

Beecher, B. (2009) 'The medical model, mental health practitioners, and individuals with schizophrenia and their families', *Journal of Social Work Practice*, vol. 23, no. 1, pp. 9–20.

Berzins, K. & Atkinson, J. (2009) 'Service users and carer's views of the Named Person provision under the Mental Health (Care and Treatment) (Scotland) Act 2003', *Journal of Mental Health*, vol. 18, no. 3, pp. 207–215.

Biestek, F. (1967) *The Casework Relationship. Fourth Impression*, George Allen and Unwin, London.

Cameron, D & McGowan, P (2013) 'The mental health social worker as a transitional participant: actively listening to 'voices' and getting into the recovery position', *Journal of Social Work Practice*, vol. 27, no. 1, pp. 21–32.

Colman, W. (1989) *On Call. The Work of a Telephone Helpline for Child Abusers*, Aberdeen University Press, Aberdeen.

Department of Health and Concordat Signatories (2014) *Mental Health Crisis Care Concordat. Improving Outcomes for People Experiencing Mental Health Crisis*, HM Government, London.

Dwyer, S. (2012) 'Walking the tightrope of a mental health act assessment', *Journal of Social Work Practice*, vol. 26, no. 1, pp. 341–353.

Gregory, M. & Thompson, A. (2013) 'From here to recovery: one service user's journey through a mental health crisis: some reflections on experience, policy and practice', *Journal of Social Work Practice*, vol. 27, no. 4, pp. 455–470.

Hardcastle M., Kennard D., Garndison S. & And Fagin L. (2007) *Experiences of Mental Health In-patient Care. Narratives from Service Users, Carers and Professionals*, Routledge, London.

Heller,T., Reynolds, J., Gomm, R., Muston, R. & Pattison, S (1996) *Mental Health Matters. A Reader*, Plagrave, Hampshire.

Hewitt, D. (2010a) 'The approved mental health professional and the nearest relative. Detention need not be negligent, even if it is unlawful', *The Journal of Adult Protection*, vol. 12, no. 4, pp. 43–45.

Hewitt, D. (2010b) 'The nearest relative: losing the right to concur?', *The Journal of Adult Protection*, vol. 12, no. 3, pp. 35–39.

Jones, R. (2013) *Mental Health Act Manual*. 16th ed. Sweet and Maxwell, London.

Laurence, J. (2003) *Pure Madness. How Fear Drives the Mental Health System*, Routledge, London.

Leff, J. (2001) *The Unbalanced Mind*, Weidenfeld and Nicolson, London.

Mayer, J. & Timms, N. (1970) *The Client Speaks: Working Class Impressions of Casework*, Routledge and Kegan Paul, London.

Nathan, J. & Webber, M. (2010) 'Mental health social work and the bureau-medicalisation of mental health care: identity in a changing world', *Journal of Social Work Practice*, vol. 24, no. 1, pp. 15–28.

Obholzer, A. & Roberts, V. (1997) *The Unconscious at Work. Individual and Organizational Stress in the Human Services*, Routledge, London.

Pilgrim, D. (2009) 'Recovery from mental health problems: scratching the surface without ethnography', *Journal of Social Work Practice*, vol. 23, no. 4, pp. 475–487.

Read, J. & Reynolds, J. (2000) *Speaking Our Minds. An Anthology*, Palgrave, Hampshire.

Rowe, D. (2003) *Depression, the Way Out of Your Prison*. 3rd ed. Routledge, London.

Ruch G., Turney D. & Ward A. (2010) *Relationship-based Practice. Getting to the Heart of Practice*, Jessica Kingsley, London.

Smith, M. (2000) 'Supervision of fear in social work. A re-evaluation of reassurance', *Journal of Social Work Practice*, vol. 14, no. 1, pp. 17–26.

Tew, J., Ramon, S., Slade, M., Bird, V., Melton, J. & Le Boutilier, C. (2012) 'Social factors and recovery from mental health difficulties: a review of the evidence', *British Journal of Social Work*, vol. 42, no. 3, pp. 443–460.

The Big Issue in the North (15–21 September 2014).

Uttarkar, V. (2010) 'An investigation into community mental health staff experiences', *Journal of Social Work Practice*, vol. 24, no. 1, pp. 49–61.

Whittaker, A. (2009) *Research Skills for Social Work*, Learning Matters, Exeter.

Wilson K., Ruch G., Lymbery M. & Cooper A. (2011) *Social Work. An Introduction to Contemporary Practice*. 2nd ed. Pearson, Edinburgh.

Winnicott, D. (1947/1987) 'Hate in the countertransference', in *Through Paediatrics to Psychoanalysis. Collected Papers*, Karnac, London.

Hanoch Yerushalmi

IMPASSES IN THE RELATIONSHIP BETWEEN THE PSYCHIATRIC REHABILITATION PRACTITIONER AND THE CONSUMER: A PSYCHODYNAMIC PERSPECTIVE

Psychiatric rehabilitation relationships can be undermined, which can potentially damage the recovery of consumers of mental health services who are coping with a prolonged serious mental illness. This might occur when practitioners who work to advance the complex rehabilitation process and need to function in diverse areas, fail to identify and respond to the unique needs involved. This might lead to a rupture in the practitioner–consumer relationship and to an impasse in the rehabilitation. In this article, an example clarifies how such an impasse can occur in a rehabilitation relationship and demonstrates the role of the practitioner in its resolution.

Social workers have occupied a central role among other helping professionals in the various areas of mental health and particularly in rehabilitation. Their broad perspective of the relationship between the individuals and their environment and their training in interpersonal communication and individual and group interventions have prepared them for the complex task of integrating persons with serious mental illness (SMI) into their community and improving their quality of life.

It is important to note that the relationship created between consumers of mental health services with SMI and the practitioners supporting them in their rehabilitation process is a crucial component on their way to recovery. Through this relationship, the practitioners can remain updated on the consumers' mental health and personal well-being, can mediate for the consumers regarding the demands and expectations of the interpersonal, economic and physical reality, and can hold ongoing dialogue and negotiation with them about their perceptions, judgments and decisions regarding their recovery directions and personal development. Consumers often use this relationship as a role model on which to develop relationships of a similar nature with significant others.

The rehabilitation relationship, just like any therapeutic or other type of relationship, is shaped by historical-relational schemas that have been instilled in each participant, and that create fantasies and expectations regarding interactions with significant others in the present. By observing their relationship, practitioners and consumers can learn about the influence of past relational experiences on the present relationship. Through this observation, consumers are able to examine, together with their rehabilitation practitioners, alternative ways of expressing their personal wishes and social needs. In addition, this key relationship and the wish to preserve it can be an important motive for consumers to persevere in realising their recovery goals, while it is clear that the consumer and the practitioner are united in the goal of the consumer's recovery. Therefore, it seems that the wholeness and continuity of the rehabilitation relationship are extremely important for the consumer's recovery and personal development. If this relationship is undermined or if there is a threat to its existence, it is essential to identify the causes and to act to resolve the ruptures that have been created.

Varied theoretical and research literature has examined impasses in therapeutic relationships involving people without SMI, as well as ways of resolving these impasses to restore the continuity of the relationship. This literature has drawn from the abundance of accumulated information and insights from the developmental psychology and self-psychology fields. These theoretical and clinical understandings are relevant also, at least to a certain extent, to relationships between practitioners and consumers in psychiatric rehabilitation. This is because these two types of relationships are based on helping empower the person receiving the help, and both aspire to advance this person's individual development. In addition, in both these types of relationships, the practitioner has greater responsibility than the consumer for its creation and preservation, despite the mutuality that might exist between them and their aspirations to equality. These two types of relationships are based on creating an atmosphere of security and on the ongoing possibility of reflective examination in order to continue the relationship, with the goal of achieving the consumer's well-being and personal growth.

In the present article, I propose to examine how the insights from the therapeutic field can be adapted to the rehabilitation relationship to cope with impasses and threats to the continuation of the relationship. These adaptations are required because of the significant differences in character, circumstance and context between these two types of helping relationships. These differences between rehabilitative and therapeutic interventions are derived largely from the unique nature of professional accompaniment in rehabilitation: using intervention strategies to help persons with SMI achieve their recovery goals and mediating between them and their social and occupational environment. These differences lead to the possibility of additional impasses in the rehabilitation relationship, but also create many opportunities for the participants' personal growth.

The article has been written in Israel, in which persons with SMI who have been examined by mental health professionals receive a "rehabilitation basket" that includes money allocated for rehabilitation purposes in the areas of supported occupation, accommodation, and leisure. Mental health professionals, primarily social workers, and also occupational therapists and experts in other disciplines, who are trained in rehabilitation intervention strategies, accompany their clients in the recovery process.

The occurrence and resolution of impasses in the therapeutic relationship

Every dyadic relationship has its own unique characteristics, which foster its participants' self-regulation and their ability to organise and make sense of their emotional reactions (Mikulincer *et al.*, 2003; Mandelbaum & Shapiro, 2011). One of the major dyadic relationship characteristics is the communication style between the two participants (Gumley *et al.*, 2008). In the mother–child dyad, for example, when the mother becomes still-faced, some children send many more signals to her and for longer periods of time than others, who quickly stop sending out signals, and independently find solutions to regulate their burning needs (Beebe & Lachmann, 1988; Morgan, 1997). Other characteristics can be expressed in ways in which the two participants in the relationship communicate their needs and mental states.

Another central characteristic of each relationship is the way its participants cope with a situation in which the congruity and harmony between them is violated, creating a threat to their relationship; also, the way in which they choose to cope with this threat and to restore the harmony to the relationship. The relationship can be mended either immediately, or slowly and in a prolonged manner through cooperation and mutuality, or in an asymmetric fashion. It is important to note that this type of dyadic relationship resolution does not usually involve merely a restoration of the previous situation, but it also includes an important developmental value for each member of the dyad, especially if they have experienced relational ruptures in their pasts. The early relational impasses occurred when the close environment was not attuned to the needs of the developing child, and did not succeed in resolving the ruptures that were created following these failures (LaMothe, 2012). Disclosing the source of these ruptures that a person has experienced and understanding how they are influencing the current ruptures will enable each member of the dyad to take a greater responsibility for interpersonal impasses that occur.

How can these relationship impasses be resolved? Psychodynamic developmental research shows that intimate relationships are regulated by internal working models (Blatt & Levy, 2003; Divino & Moore, 2010; Beebe *et al.*, 2012), which exist in the minds of each member of the dyad. These models clarify for the person what motivates the people in his or her environment to act, and through these models he or she knows their mind. These models enable the person to create a plan of action to resolve a deteriorating relationship with another person (Lyons-Ruth, 1999).

The best place to foster the ability to develop these models about the minds of others and simultaneously to learn about their models is in psychotherapy. A therapist–patient relationship evolves through continuous but non-linear movement of 'matches, mismatches, ruptures, and repair' (Stern *et al.*, 1998, p. 302). Joint therapist–patient observation of their interaction can develop an important mental skill that will assist patients to resolve relational impasses with significant others and help advance their interpersonal goals. The therapeutic relationship is not only a safe, protected relationship that includes continued investigative dialogue. By virtue of his or her training, the therapist is highly skilled in knowing the patient's mind as well as in the use of reflection to understand complex interpersonal processes that occur in therapy.

Therapists always play a central role in managing relational impasses in the therapeutic interaction. They must include the patient in the investigation to clarify how the therapist failed empathically, which led to a rupture in the relationship; in other words, to identify which of the patient's psychological needs the therapist disregarded because of insufficient empathy with the patient's experience (Kohut, 1984; Herzig, 2001; Kitron, 2003; Silverberg, 2011). This disregard of the patient's needs as a result of the therapist's lack of full and appropriate attunement to the patient can lead to traumatic ruptures in the therapeutic relationship, which reconstruct similar failures of parental figures in the patient's past. These past failures created negative relational expectations in the patient, who, to prevent their recurrence, would often adopt behaviours such as avoidance, excessive self-protection, antagonism, withdrawal into the self and inflexibility. Therapists and patients must explore and understand their mutual reactions, which were based on negative expectations from their pasts, which invaded the therapeutic relationship.

Good management of a relational impasse is achieved only when therapists take responsibility and acknowledge their empathic failure to patients. Only then can patients also take similar responsibility for their own contribution to the development of the relational impasse. If this clarification succeeds, their relationship can include much more affection, admiration, sense of like-mindedness and mutual comfort in the future. The successful resolve of relationships creates similar relational experiences and positive expectations in patients, which will enrich their lives (Lichtenberg, 2003). Resolving these impasses in the therapeutic relationship empowers both participants' sense of trustworthiness and security, increases the sense of resiliency of their self-experience and strengthens their self-image. It also improves the patients' belief in their own ability to resolve ruptured relationships when they identify with the skills and strategies used by the therapists to manage empathic failures. Hence, the patients learn to internalise essential, healthy aspects of the therapist's character (LaMothe, 2012).

The occurrence and resolution of impasses in the rehabilitation relationship

The psychiatric rehabilitation literature gives supreme importance to the quality of the rehabilitation relationship that respects consumers and is tailored to their needs and aspirations (Deegan, 1990; Anthony et al., 2003; Finaret & Shor, 2006; McGuire-Snieckus et al., 2007; Bishop, 2012). This relationship serves as the foundation and focal point of support in the recovery process, in which consumers struggle to attain an enriching, meaningful life, in which they are the shaping agents of their environment (Baumeister & Vohs, 2002; Davidson, 2007). The existence of a strong rehabilitation relationship requires a highly skilled practitioner, but first and foremost is evidence of the consumer's profound willingness to cooperate on this difficult and complex path.

Consumers' first-hand evidence describes the centrality of their relationship with the practitioner, and the extent to which it has a decisive influence on advancing the recovery process. Conversely, it also shows how the relationship can seriously impede the recovery process, can damage consumers' self-esteem and can lead to a sense of helplessness, humiliation, apathy and despair (Deegan, 1990; Anthony et al., 2003; Browne et al., 2012). Therefore, it is very important to examine, as investigated in psychotherapy, how ruptures are created in the rehabilitation relationship and how they can be resolved. This investigation can have important implications for practitioners' and consumers' expectations of these relationships and for their motivation to continue and struggle for their advancement. To examine this subject and its significance for rehabilitation, we must first point to several unique aspects of the rehabilitation relationship, which influence its character and development.

a. According to the World Health Organization (WHO), rehabilitation of people with disabilities, including psychiatric disability, is a process designed to enable them to achieve their highest potential in physical, sensory, intellectual, psychological and social functions (WHO, 2011). This requires the combined effort of various authorities in the community, which deal with education, medicine, religious services, and more, each contributing its part to the rehabilitation and recovery process. The practitioner–consumer relationship is only one of a variety of relationships that need to be coped with in the community and the mental health services. This fact influences the nature and the development of this relationship, even if it is the most central or most important among them.

   The large number of therapeutic authorities sometimes creates splits among them. These splits might cause consumers either to idealise one of the supporting figures in the rehabilitation process or to perceive him or her as excessively harmful (Kernberg, 1975; Akhtar, 1998; Cavalli, 2010). These types of splits might complicate or delay the rehabilitation process, mainly when there is no ongoing communication between the different supporting authorities. On the other hand, in the case of cooperation and links between the helping and support authorities, their multiplicity and diversity can facilitate integrative and intensive rehabilitation activity, which covers many and varied areas of the consumer's life.

b. Psychiatric rehabilitation usually continues for a relatively prolonged period and the professional task of the practitioner is more multi-disciplinary than in therapy. As well as therapeutic intervention, it includes ongoing preventive intervention and greater accessibility of the community services (Hughes, 1994; McCabe & Priebe, 2004). In addition, this professional task includes ongoing coping with social stigma directed towards consumers, which might cause them distress, reduce their mental well-being, lead to low self-esteem and self-efficacy and decrease the likelihood of recovery (Link, 2001; Corrigan & Watson, 2002; Dinos et al., 2004).

   It is important to note that because of this diversity of tasks, rehabilitation practitioners are forced to manage their professional encounters with consumers in many different locations, such as a closed ward in a psychiatric hospital, a community mental health centre, various rehabilitation frameworks (employment, study, etc.), in the home of the consumer with a psychiatric disorder, and so on. This lack of permanence undoubtedly has an impact on the development, character, and durability of the rehabilitation relationship.

c. Consumers often enter the rehabilitation relationship in a far more weakened state than patients in psychotherapy that is not part of a recovery journey from SMI. This depends on the traumatic history of the attacks of the illness and of social and institutional harm to these consumers. This problematic history might cause personal distress to many consumers and harm their social and occupational functioning. All these might lead consumers to adopt passive stances of dependence, which cause difficulties when providing help, rehabilitation services and support for these consumers (Nath et al., 2012).

These characteristics of the rehabilitation relationship might fatigue the practitioners, who are required to be present and responsive far beyond the time allocated in the regular sessions. Moreover, sometimes, they create negative stances because of burnout resulting from the daily encounter with multiple problems and needs and because practitioners perceive rehabilitative work as unrewarding and lacking in professional prestige (Anthony, 1993; Russinova et al., 2006).

d. Despite the aim of creating a supportive, recovery-oriented rehabilitation system for consumers, which is accompanied by a good professional relationship, it is difficult for practitioners and their consumers to agree on the goals of the professional process, unlike in the therapeutic relationship. A study on the subject clarified that because of the large gap in the practitioners' and consumers' perceptions of the rehabilitation goals, in most cases it was the practitioners who made the final decisions for their consumers. These included the nature of medication, participation in a group, etc. The consumers themselves made the decisions only in a small number of cases, and in even fewer cases, the decisions were made jointly by both sides (Matthias et al., 2012). This state of affairs places a heavy responsibility on the practitioners, and further reduces the balance between practitioners and consumers.

The possibilities for developing an empathic failure in the rehabilitation relationship, which is so important for the recovery process, are linked to the many areas of interaction between consumers and rehabilitation practitioners, and in the varied challenges mentioned here. In this way, many relational ruptures can develop when one of the rehabilitation relationship channels does not receive appropriate attention from the practitioner. This occurs through the practitioner's lack of alertness leading to a disregard of the consumer's needs. Such an empathic failure might constitute a reconstruction of many previous bitter failures of the environment to respond to the consumer's diverse and complex needs.

In the following section, I bring an example of an undermined rehabilitation relationship between practitioner and consumer. Even though the undermining was the result of external events, the rupture occurred mainly because of the practitioner's lack of sensitivity in her reaction to these events. Similar stories may be told by other practitioners working in this field, who have to cope with relational impasses in the rehabilitation relationship.

Example

Tom is a 34-year-old rehabilitation consumer who has experienced psychiatric hospitalisations in his past, including one particularly traumatic case. This was when he was hospitalised by force and the event has left him with psychological scars. He has also been in trouble with the law, having had a tendency to become inebriated from time to time and to start fights with people around him. Today, however, he is emotionally and functionally balanced and a long time has passed since his last hospitalisation and criminal arrest. For a considerable period, he has been in supported employment in a store selling candy and snacks, which is managed like any other commercial business. As part of their rehabilitation process, the consumers who work in this store sell high-quality products to prepare them for inclusion in the unsupported business sector.

Tom has recently been promoted to the position of shift manager, and is responsible for other consumers employed in the store. Most of the time, the consumers function relatively well on both the personal and social levels, and serve the store's regular and occasional customers. As shift manager, Tom manages the cash register independently and makes sure that other consumers working under him on the same shift deal appropriately with customers' payments. Tom succeeds in coping with many difficulties that periodically arise and functions well in his shift manager role. He knows when to call the rehabilitation worker in charge of running the store for advice on how to act.

Tom has a good relationship with his rehabilitation practitioner, who provides individual support in his occupational development and with his coping on a social and family level. Together with Tom, the practitioner examines the difficulties in his social and occupational tasks on an ongoing basis. They weigh up possibilities of how to cope with them and plan future procedures together. The rehabilitation practitioner makes sure to give gradually more space to Tom's opinion, and little by little tries to reduce her authoritative intervention. In this way, she helps him to build and establish his interpersonal, management and business capabilities, while serving as a clearer and more stable figure than family figures in his past. Several times during his encounters with the rehabilitation practitioner, Tom expresses anger towards her for not always being present when disagreements occur with other consumers working in the store, and for not automatically taking his side in these events. When she investigates how and why he has reacted impulsively to these events, without giving his response enough consideration, he feels hurt and abandoned by her. The rehabilitation practitioner usually succeeds in quelling Tom's anger during their sessions, without reacting in a hurtful way, and Tom continues to perceive her as a positive figure.

After about a year in this job in the store, staff members begin to notice that sums of money are going missing from the cash register. They believe that one of the rehabilitation consumers employed in the store is taking the money, but cannot be sure about this and acknowledge that mistakes might have been made when recording revenues and expenses. They ask Tom and the other consumers to be extra careful to be precise when dealing with the money, but Tom appears to be deeply offended by the request itself. After some time, Tom manages to calm down so as not to explode and act on impulse. When the subject arises, he is soothed by the rehabilitation practitioner's emotion regulation and mediation of the reality and its meaning for him. However, some time later, an incident occurs that threatens critical damage to Tom's progress and the rehabilitation relationship.

The rehabilitation staff and the consumers discover an apparent break-in to the store, when a significant sum of money and several items of stock have disappeared. However, the lock at the entrance to the store has not been broken and the offenders seem not to have used burglary equipment to break in, but someone has used a key to open the door. These circumstances arouse the staff members' suspicion that the theft has been committed by an employee who carries a key to the store. The significance of these indirect and implicit accusations by the rehabilitation service administration and the staff members is that one of the store employees is responsible for the theft. They all become suspects, despite having declared that they had nothing to do with the incident. Following a discussion among the rehabilitation service staff, it is decided that, from now on, two people (rather than one) will be responsible for opening the store, to prevent additional theft.

It is clear from Tom's facial expression and reactions that he is exceedingly alarmed by everything that has occurred. He seems to be interpreting the staff members' suspicions as a deep, personal affront, and reacts with anxiety. He withdraws into himself, remains continually silent and escapes back home as soon as he can. After spending several days at home and not coming to work, the rehabilitation practitioner telephones him. In this conversation, Tom informs her of his wish to leave the rehabilitation framework and states that he is ending this contact as a furious protest against the staff members' unfounded and incriminating accusations against him. The rehabilitation practitioner, who knows how important the occupational framework is for him and for his rehabilitation process, which is progressing so well, pleads with him not to leave the framework in the absence of an alternative arrangement. Tom does not listen, however, and attends neither meetings nor his work shifts in the days following the event, and neither does he answer telephone calls at home. The rehabilitation practitioner makes investigations on his behalf as to the existence of alternative frameworks, in the event that one would be needed, and consults the other staff members as to how she should act at this critical stage of his rehabilitation.

The rehabilitation practitioner waits until the rehabilitation consumers' payday to make contact with Tom once again. She telephones him, and as soon as he answers, asks to meet him to pay him his wages, to see how he is, and to assess how to proceed with the rehabilitation relationship. At first, Tom refuses to meet her, but later, he agrees, and when they finally do meet, he tells her that he feels very isolated and angry and that he has turned once again to alcohol to calm himself down, as in the past. The drinking from which he has abstained for so long is causing him states of anxiety and troublesome thoughts, which intensify his emotional state and unrest. He senses despair and helplessness, and does not believe that he will ever be able to return to such good, well-organised employment. He tells the rehabilitation practitioner that he has not applied to any other framework and that his family feels helpless and is just as alarmed as he is, as was the case in previous distress situations.

The rehabilitation practitioner states clearly to Tom that she now understands that she made an error of judgment. When the theft occurred, she had not immediately understood that Tom was likely to feel accused, and she now realises that she should have protected him from any type of overt or covert accusations. She also admits that she erred in allowing several days to pass before insisting on renewing their communication so that she could intervene and help him through the current crisis. She says that she had incorrectly evaluated Tom's degree of sensitivity when confronted with such accusations and the extent of his trauma in relation to a criminal act and potential trouble with the police. She also reassures Tom that neither the rehabilitation administration nor the staff has made any official complaint to the police, and that until such a step has been taken, Tom is at no actual risk of being questioned or accused of the theft.

Tom is very relieved after hearing the practitioner's clarifications, as anxiety impairs his ability to distinguish between a general, unfounded suspicion and an open accusation, which might lead to a criminal investigation and trial. In this conversation, it becomes clear that Tom has already imagined that he is pursued and attacked by the police, that he will undoubtedly be brought to trial in the near future, and will eventually find himself behind bars. These imaginings have aroused traumatic memories of situations of helplessness and loneliness, when he felt as if no-one in the world could understand or rescue him. He senses great relief on hearing the rehabilitation practitioner's clarifications regarding possible and real dangers, as well as by her admitting to misjudging his reactions and needs, and to her mishandling of the entire event. He is relieved to understand that he is not alone in being at risk of making errors of judgment, but that even the rehabilitation practitioner, whom he perceives as strong and experienced, is not immune from mistakes.

The rehabilitation practitioner proposes that they can now understand the degree to which Tom's reaction of alarm was caused by anxiety, when he disappeared from his work in the store and stopped communicating with her. She promises Tom that she will explain his position to the person in charge of the rehabilitation service and that she is sure that he will also make an effort to protect him. She suggests that Tom arrange a consultation with his physician to consider changing his medication to deal with his current state of agitation and to help him regain emotional balance and intact social-occupational functioning. She also promises to meet with his family to give them strength and guidance regarding how to help Tom, and that as soon as he feels ready to return to work, she will accompany him to the store. At the end of their conversation, the rehabilitation practitioner accompanies Tom to the bus stop on his journey home. Following their meeting, she initiates several conversations with the members of the rehabilitation staff, with the head of the rehabilitation service, with Tom's physician and with his family. She explains to them about his current difficulties and they examine together how they can attempt to restore balance in Tom's life and in his path to recovery.

This example illustrates how an impasse with traumatic components occurred in the consumer's path to recovery. This impasse led to problematic functioning, such as impairing his judgment of reality as well as his ability to regulate his anxiety. Consequently, the consumer regressed from important rehabilitative achievements and lapsed into problematic coping patterns from the past, which put his continued employment and longstanding relationship with the rehabilitation practitioner at risk. These non-adaptive coping patterns from the past included drinking alcohol and social withdrawal, while experiencing great emotional distress and considerable damage to his sense of self-worth. In addition, his sense of reality and ongoing ability for reality testing were noticeably damaged, which caused him to feel very lonely and fearful.

It is very likely that the consumer's sense of isolation, his regression to previous problematic patterns and the damaging effects of the alcohol reduced his ability to organise and deal with both the external and internal reality in an appropriate and logical manner. He may have found himself plagued by haunting visions, which increased his sense of threat and personal crisis. It is possible that, at these moments, he was reconstructing the memory of the traumatic experience of forceful hospitalisation, when he had felt helpless and the victim of a violent act. This is because people who have experienced trauma become more sensitive to stimuli that remind them of the traumatic event. These stimuli apparently played a part in his escape and disconnection from his self-experience by drinking alcohol, which temporarily distances genuine worries and provides a false sense of security and calm. In addition, the consumer temporarily lost his ability to distinguish between a remote suspicion and an actual accusation, or even between others' wish to harm him or to take revenge on him, despite his innocence. Additional anxiety was aroused because of his increasing need and dependence on external assistance, which threatened his independence and autonomy. It was particularly in this situation of need and distress that the consumer experienced an empathic failure on the part of the rehabilitation practitioner, who did not succeed in the early identification of the intensity of his experience and the greatness of his need.

Conclusions

Social workers who work as practitioners in mental health rehabilitation have a good understanding of the importance of a harmonious and mutual client–practitioner relationship. As in other areas of individual and group work, for the benefit of the consumers in the mental health services, the practitioners need to devote attention and emotional investment to preserving and strengthening the professional relationship with their clients. Through considering relevant literature in other, similar areas of professional help and through considering the specific characteristics of the mental health rehabilitation, several conclusions can be reached. The event described in the example is characteristic of many similar cases, both more and less dramatic, of a rupture in the consumer's relationship with the rehabilitation community and the rehabilitation practitioner. In these cases, it is necessary to seek ways to restore and strengthen the relationship, and even to grow from the rupture. In the following paragraphs, I suggest several conclusions that can be derived from this typical example and point to three types of empathic failures that are characteristic of the rehabilitation relationship, in addition to those that exist in the therapeutic relationship.

a. The failure to identify the consumer's need to strengthen his or her perception of reality is characteristic of the rehabilitation relationship but does not appear in a similar way in the therapeutic relationship. The need to strengthen the perception of reality usually appears in children, who have not yet established their ability for level-headed coping with reality and who are in need of the adults' perception of reality. However, this perception might be elusive also for consumers because of pathological processes: psychiatric symptoms, especially those related to active psychosis, might impair their normal perception of reality and create illusions of an alternative reality. Therefore, rehabilitation practitioners need to be continually sensitive to the consumer's needs of reality assessment, which might be strengthened or weakened in accordance with the development of pathological processes or with changes in the rehabilitation or family environment. Practitioners sometimes fail to identify these needs, which might cause distress to the consumers because they lose confidence in their reality testing. This might cause difficulty with the consumers' ongoing task of separating the external and internal worlds, which is a task that all people face, but is more difficult for people with SMI (Greenacre, 1973).

b. Failure to protect consumers from being the target of hostility from the social environment because of their eccentricities and because they violate or threaten to violate social and cultural rules. Many studies have exposed this hostility towards consumers, which is manifest in a persistent social stigma, which has implications for the consumers' lives: the sense of distress, reduced psychological well-being, low self-esteem and self-efficacy and a general decrease in the likelihood of recovery (Link, 2001; Corrigan & Watson, 2002; Dinos *et al.*, 2004).

c. Hostility towards consumers might be expressed by family members, in the workplace or in the community in which they live. This can cast a shadow on the consumer's relationship with the practitioner, if he or she does not succeed in identifying and protecting the consumer from it. However, practitioners might overlook the hostility of the environment towards consumers because of their own difficulties or feelings of helplessness or despair during the rehabilitation process.

d. Failure to identify the consumers' need to depend on the rehabilitation practitioners, which lead to regressive states during their rehabilitation. It must be explained that this regression is a return to functioning that characterised the person's previous periods of immaturity, includes a childish attitude to the other and stands in contrast to adult functioning, to growth and individuation. Therefore, regression might actually cause an increase in mental and social disability and stagnation both inside and outside the rehabilitation process (Moore & Fine, 1990; Coen, 2000). The consumers' need for dependence on the rehabilitation practitioner is usually greater in comparison to psychotherapy patients. This is because of their psychiatric disability and their need for the practitioner's constant mediation between themselves and their social and institutional environment. Disregard of these needs might cause consumers to feel lonely and anxious.

On the other hand, the rehabilitation practitioners might have difficulty in identifying different types of needs among consumers—of separation-individuation (Mahler *et al.*, 1975), which might arise specifically because of the anxiety caused by the need for dependence and the wish for regression. These needs are expressed in the wish for autonomy, for independent decision-making and for personal responsibility. The failure of rehabilitation practitioners to identify these needs might cause consumers to feel misunderstood and belittled, and might harm their motivation for recovery, thus hindering the possibility for harmonious cooperation.

The appearance and resolution of these unique failures that are typical to the rehabilitation relationship increase the risk of a rupture in the consumers' rehabilitation and recovery process. Nevertheless, there is no doubt that if practitioners acknowledge these failures and take responsibility for their ability to identify and react to the consumers' needs, this can greatly advance the rehabilitation relationship and the recovery process. The practitioners' recognition of this responsibility can validate the consumers' feelings and their perception of their interpersonal reality. Moreover, it can serve as a model for the consumers for reflection on interpersonal events in which they play a part and for taking appropriate personal responsibility, which would advance their relationships and personal growth.

References

Akhtar, S. (1998) 'From simplicity through contradiction to paradox: the evolving psychic reality of the borderline patient in treatment', *International Journal of Psycho-Analysis*, vol. 79, pp. 241–252.

Anthony, W. A. (1993) 'Recovery from mental illness: the guiding vision of the mental health system in the 1990s', *Innovations and Research*, vol. 2, pp. 17–24.

Anthony, W. A., Rogers, E. S. & Farkas, M. D. (2003) 'Research on evidence-based practices: future directions in an era of recovery', *Community Mental Health Journal*, vol. 39, pp. 101–114.

Baumeister, R. F. & Vohs, K. D. (2002) 'The pursuit of meaningfulness', in *Handbook of Positive Psychology*, eds C. R. Snyder & S. J. Lopez, Oxford Press, London, pp. 608–618.

Beebe, B. & Lachmann, F. (1988) 'The contribution of mother-infant mutual influence to the origins of self and object representations', *Psychoanalytic Psychology*, vol. 5, pp. 350–337.

Beebe, B., Lachmann, F., Markese, S. & Bahrick, L. (2012) 'On the origins of disorganized attachment and internal working models', *Psychoanalytic Dialogues*, vol. 22, no. 2, pp. 253–272.

Bishop, M. (2012) 'Quality of life and psychosocial adaptation to chronic illness and acquired disability: a conceptual and theoretical synthesis', in *Psychological and Social Impact of Illness and Disability*, eds M. Irmo & M. Stebnicki, Springer, New York, pp. 179–191.

Blatt, S. J. & Levy, K. N. (2003) 'Attachment theory, psychoanalysis, personality development, and psychopathology', *Psychoanalytic Inquiry*, vol. 23, pp. 102–150.

Browne, G., Cashin, A. & Graham, I. (2012) 'The therapeutic relationship and mental health nursing: it is time to articulate what we do!', *Journal of Psychiatric and Mental Health Nursing*, vol. 19, no. 9, pp. 839–843.

Cavalli, A. (2010) 'Primal splitting as a basis for emotional and cognitive development in children', *Journal of Analytical Psychology*, vol. 55, pp. 601–602.

Coen, S. J. (2000) 'The wish to regress in patient and analyst', *Journal of the American Psychoanalytic Association*, vol. 48, pp. 785–810.

Corrigan, P. W. & Watson, A. C. (2002) 'The paradox of self-stigma and mental illness', *Clinical Psychology: Science and Practice*, vol. 9, no. 1, pp. 35–53.

Davidson, L. (2007) 'Habits and other anchors of everyday life that people with psychiatric disabilities may not take for granted', *OTJR: Occupation, Participation and Health*, vol. 27, no. suppl. 1, pp. 60–68.

Deegan, P. (1990) 'Spirit breaking: when the helping professions hurt', *Humanistic Psychologist*, vol. 18, no. 3, pp. 301–313.

Dinos, S., Stevens, S., Serfaty, M., Weich, S. & King, M. (2004) 'Stigma: the feelings and experiences of 46 people with mental illness', *British Journal of Psychiatry*, vol. 184, pp. 176–181.

Divino, C. L. & Moore, M. S. (2010) 'Integrating neurobiological findings into psychodynamic psychotherapy training and practice', *Psychoanalytic Dialogues*, vol. 20, pp. 337–355.

Finaret, A. E. & Shor, R. (2006) 'Perceptions of professionals about the nature of rehabilitation relationships with persons with mental illness and the dilemmas and conflicts that characterize these relationships', *Qualitative Social Work*, vol. 5, no. 2, pp. 151–166.

Greenacre, P. (1973) 'The primal scene and the sense of reality', *Psychoanalytic Quarterly*, vol. 42, pp. 10–41.

Gumley, A., Schwannauer, M., MacBeth, A. & Read, J. (2008) 'Emotional recovery and staying well after psychosis: an attachment-based conceptualization', *Attachment: New Direction in Psychotherapy and Related Psychoanalysis Journal*, vol. 2, pp. 127–148.

Herzig, C. (2001) 'Good breast/bad analyst: false dichotomies in understanding aggressive patients', *Fort Da*, vol. 7, pp. 56–78.

Hughes, R. (1994) 'Psychiatric rehabilitation: an essential health service for people with serious and persistent mental illness', in *An Introduction to Psychiatric Rehabilitation*, ed. The Publication Committee of I.A.P.S.R.S, I.A.P.S.R.S Publications, New York, pp. 9–17.

Kernberg, O. (1975) *Borderline Conditions and Pathological Narcissism*, Aronson, New York.

Kitron, D. G. (2003) 'Repetition compulsion and self-psychology', *International Journal of Psycho-Analysis*, vol. 84, pp. 427–441.

Kohut, H. (1984) *How Does Analysis Cure?*, University of Chicago Press, Chicago.

LaMothe, R. (2012) 'Potential space: creativity, resistance, and resiliency in the face of racism', *Psychoanalytic Review*, vol. 99, pp. 851–876.

Lichtenberg, J. (2003) 'A clinician's view of attachment theory and research', *Psychoanalytic Inquiry*, vol. 23, pp. 151–206.

Link, B. (2001) 'Stigma as a barrier to recovery: the consequences of stigma for the self-esteem of people with mental illness', *Psychiatric Services*, vol. 52, pp. 1621–1626.

Lyons-Ruth, K. (1999) 'The two-person unconscious', *Psychoanalytic Inquiry*, vol. 19, pp. 576–617.

Mahler, M., Pine, F. & Bergman, A. (1975) *The Psychological Birth of the Human Infant*, New York, Basic Books.

Mandelbaum, T. & Shapiro, J. (2011) 'Being psychologically held: separation and reparation in the parent-child relationship', *Psychoanalytic Social Work*, vol. 18, pp. 54–78.

Matthias, M. S., Salyers, M. P., Rollins, A. L. & Frankel, R. M. (2012) 'Decision making in recovery-oriented mental health care', *Psychiatric Rehabilitation Journal*, vol. 35, no. 4, pp. 305–314.

McCabe, R. & Priebe, S. (2004) 'The therapeutic relationship in the treatment of severe mental illness: a review of methods and findings', *International Journal of Social Psychiatry*, vol. 50, no. 2, pp. 115–128.

Mcguire-Snieckus, R., Mccabe, R., Catty, J., Hansson, L. & Priebei, S. (2007) 'A new scale to assess the therapeutic relationship in community mental health care: STAR', *Psychological Medicine*, vol. 37, pp. 85–95.

Mikulincer, M., Shaver, P. R. & Pereg, D. (2003) 'Attachment theory and affect regulation: the dynamics, development, and cognitive consequences of attachment-related strategies', *Motivation and Emotion*, vol. 27, no. 2, pp. 77–102.

Moore B. E. & Fine B. D. (1990) *Psychoanalytic Terms and Concepts*, American Psychoanalytic Association and Yale University Press, New Haven.

Morgan, A. C. (1997) 'The application of infant research to psychoanalytic theory and therapy', *Psychoanalytic Psychology*, vol. 14, pp. 315–336.

Nath, S. B., Alexander, L. B. & Solomon, P. L. (2012) 'Case managers' perspectives on the therapeutic alliance: a qualitative study', *Social Psychiatry and Psychiatric Epidemiology*, vol. 74, pp. 1815–1826.

Russinova, Z., Rogers, E. S. & Ellison, M. L. (2006) *Recovery-Promoting Relationships Scale* (Manual), Center for Psychiatric Rehabilitation, Boston.

Silverberg, F. (2011) 'The Tao of self psychology: was Heinz Kohut a Taoist sage?', *Psychoanalytic Inquiry*, vol. 31, pp. 475–488.

Stern, D. N., Sander, L. W., Nahum, J. P., Lyon-Ruth, K., Morgan, C., Bruschweilerstern, N. & Tronick, E. Z. (1998) 'Dyadically expanded states of consciousness and the process of therapeutic change', *Infant Mental Health Journal*, vol. 19, pp. 300–308.

WHO (World Health Organization) (2011) *World Report on Disability*, Geneva, WHO Press.

Index

Note: Page numbers in **bold** type refer to figures
Page numbers in *italic* type refer to tables

abuse: physical and sexual 74; schools 74; trauma 25; violence 75
academic scores 27
adult onset (AOS) 24
adults 27
Alianait Mental Wellness Action Plan 81
antipsychotic medication: youths 26
arrest rates 55
Atkinson, K.: and Berzins, K. 94
Audla, T. 85
Australian university 11; Social Work Field Education Unit 11–13
awareness: trauma 14

Barns, A. 46
behaviour 47; emotional characteristics 24–5
Berzins, K.: and Atkinson, K. 94
Biestek, F. 103
Bishop, S.R.: *et al.* 9–10
Blueprint for Life 76
body image: women 56
body image disorder (BID) 45–6
body weight management 43
Bordo, S. 45
Brown, C.G.: *et al.* 43, 45, 46, 47
building resilience 79–80, 86
bullying 32
Burr, V. 44, 46

Cahill, A.J. 47
Cameron, D.: and McGowan, P. 94
Canada 84; Chief Public Health Officer 74; children 54; government 78; indigenous peoples 74; mental health services 56; Pauktuutit Inuit Women 76; youths 54
Cannon, M.: *et al.* 27
caregiver: support networks 30; youths 29–30
Centre for Contemplative Mind in Society: Tree of Contemplative Practice 12–13, **12**
Chandler, S.: and Jones, J.B. 43

Chen, Y.-L.: *et al.* 3, 23–38
Chief Public Health Officer: Canada 74
childhood onset (COS) 24, 27
children 83; police encounters 53–72; psychotic symptoms 23; severe emotional disturbances (SEDs) 27; and siblings conflict 58–61; United States 23
Clandinin, D.J.: and Connelly, F.M. 9, 10–11, 13, 14, 18, 20
Client Speaks, The, social work study 95–6
climate change 84
cognitive behavioural therapy (CBT) 38, 40, 42–9
cognitive-behavioural approaches 30, 32
colonial relations: Tester and McNicoll on 75
colonisation 78, 84
communication: Approved Mental Health Professional (AHMP) 100; individual educational plans (IEPs) 31–2
community: elders 81–2; health 83; marginalised 85; youth 81–2
community-based mental health services 55, 56
confessional mode 44
conflict: children and siblings 58–61
Connelly, F.M.: and Clandinin, D.J. 9, 10–11, 13, 14, 18, 20
constructed knowledge space: Healy on 10–11
consumer 45; hostility towards 117; modern 45; need 116, 117; protection 116; psychiatric rehabilitation practitioner 107–20
Cresswell, J.W.: and Ollerenshaw, J.A. 14
criminalisation 54, 55, 62–4
Crofford, R.: *et al.* 3, 23–38
Crooks, C.: and Morris, M. 4, 73–90
cultural identity 79
culture 45

delusions 24–5, 28, 29, 30, 32
depression 25
DeRosse, P.: *et al.* 25
Diagnostic and Statistical Manual of Mental Disorders (DSM II) 24

disability 111
disciplinary power 44
discourses 18
docile bodies 44, 45–6
Dwyer, S. 93

economic status 96
elders: community 81–2
emotional characteristics: behaviours 24–5
employees 80
ethical practice 17–19
ethical problems 99
Ethics Approval 11

family: support networks 30–1; violence 61
feedback: individual educational plans (IEPs) 31;
    service users 95; *TripAdvisor* 95
feelings: sharing 82
female body image: therapy 39–52
Fenstermacher, G.D. 8, 9
finance management 30–1
Food and Drug Administration (FDA) 29
Foote, C.: and Franke, A.W. 39, 40
Furlotte, C.: and Hick, S.F. 9

generalisations 57
genetic vulnerability 25–6
Gibson, M. 3, 39–52
governmentality 43–4
Greenberg, J.L.: and Wilhelm, S. 40
Gregor, C. 5
Gregory, M.: and Thompson, A. 94

hallucinations 24, 25, 28, 29–30
Hanh, T.N. 7
Hardcastle, M.: *et al.* 96, 97, 101
health: community 83; indigenous organisations 84;
    wellness 9
Healy, K. 8, 9, 10, 11, 16, 18, 19
Heaney, S.: *Squarings* 2
Hick, S.F.: and Furlotte, C. 9
Hohman, B.: *Motivational Interviewing in Social Work
    Practice* 5
hospitalisations 31
human beings 103
Human Rights Act (1993) 93

identity: cultural 79
imagery: intrusive 61
individual educational plans (IEPs) 28, 31–2;
    communication 31–2; feedback 31
individualisation 41–2
Individuals with Disability Educational Act (IDEA,
    2004) 27
insurance: United States 30
internalisation 86
International Statistical Classification of Diseases and
    Related Health Problems (ICS) 24

intervention 62
intrusive imagery 61
Inuit Tapiriit Kanatami (ITK) 76
Irving, A. 46

Jaswal, P.: and Liegghio, M. 3, 53–72
Jones, J.B.: and Chandler, S. 43
Jones, R. 92, 93

Kamatsiaqtut Help Line 76
Keenan, E.K. 44, 46
Kim-Cohen, J.: *et al.* 25
Kirmayer, L.J.: *et al.* 74
knowledge 8, 9, 10, 18; creation 19–20; cultural
    identity 79; professional 8
Koprowska, J. 5
Kral, M.J.: *et al.* 81

language 45
Liegghio, M.: *et al.* 55–6; and Jaswal, P. 3, 53–72
literature review 54–6
Lynn, R.: and Mensinga, J. 3, 7–22

McGowan, P.: and Cameron, D. 94
McNicoll, P.: and Tester, F.J. 75
Malmgren, K.: and Meisel, S. 27
Manning, A.: *et al.* 3, 23–38
Markula, P. 40, 41–2, 44, 45
medical discourse 47
medicalisation 43
medication: antipsychotic 26; assessing impact 28–9;
    Food and Drug Administration 29
Meisel, S.: and Malmgren, K. 27
Mensinga, J.: and Lynn, R. 3, 7–22
Mental Health Act (MHA, 1983) 91–106
mental health rehabilitation: social workers 116
mental health services: Canada 56; community-based
    55, 56
Miller, W.R.: and Rollnick, S. 5
modern consumer 45
Moffatt, K. 42
Morris, M.: and Crooks, C. 4, 73–90
Motivational Interviewing (Miller and Rollnick) 5
Motivational Interviewing in Social Work Practice
    (Hohman) 5

Nathan, J.: and Webber, M. 94
National Aboriginal Health Organisation (NAHO)
    76
National Alliance for Mental Health Illness (NAMI)
    32
National Heart Lung and Blood Institute (USA) 43
National Inuit Youth Council (NIYC) 76
National Strategy on Inuit Education 80
need: consumer 116, 117
negotiated practice 16–17
Nunavut Suicide Prevention Strategy Action Plan (2011)
    77

observation: therapeutic relationship 109
Odgers, C.: *et al.* 55
Olfson, M.: *et al.* 24
Ollerenshaw, J.A.: and Cresswell, J.W. 14
onset: adult (AO) 24; childhood (COS) 24, 27; chronic 25; insidious 25; youth 25–6
Out of Hours: Approved Mental Health Professional (AHMP) 100

parenting: relationship skills 83
Pauktuutit Inuit Women of Canada 76, 82
Phillips, C. 42, 44
physical abuse 74
physical restraint 55
Pilgrim, D. 94
power 39, 49; disciplinary 44; inequity 44; reflection 46
practitioner narratives: individual participant stories 14
priority: realities 83–4
professional development workshop 11
professional learning networks (PLNs) 32
professionalism 19
protection: consumer 116
psychotic symptomology 26
psychotic symptoms: children 23

Read, J.: and Reynolds, J. 95, 98, 103
realities: priority 83–4
reflection 46
rehabilitation 116; consumer example 112–16
relationship skills: parenting 83
relatives: nearest 91–106
resistance 47
restraint: physical 55
Reynolds, J.: and Read, J. 95, 98, 103
Rittner, B.: *et al.* 3, 23–38
Robst, J.: *et al.* 55
Rollnick, S.: and Miller, W.R. 5

safety plans: violence 61
school 78, 83; abuse 74; outcomes 27
serious mental illness (SMI) 107, 108
service user: buzz words 96; experience 96–7; feedback 95; perspective 96; review 96, 96–8
services 27–8; control of 80; United States 27–8
severe emotional disturbances (SEDs) 27
sexual abuse 74
sharing feelings: speaking out 82
Smith, M.S. 4, 91–106

social construct 14–16
social work: practice 39–52
Social Work Field Education Unit: Australian university 11–13
social worker: mental health rehabilitation 116
speaking out 82
stigmatisation 54, 62–4; research 56–7
support networks: caregivers 30; family 30–1
surveillance 42, 42–3, 49

teaching 8, 10–11
technologies of the self 41–2
Tester, F.J.: and McNicoll, P. 75
Tew, J.: *et al.* 93, 96
theraputic authorities 111
theraputic relationship 109–10; intimate 109; observation 109
therapy: female body image 39–52
Thompson, A.: and Gregory, M. 94
three dimensional space approach 9, 14, 18
trauma: and abuse 25; awareness 14
Tree of Contemplative Practice 12–13, **12**
Tretheway, A. 42
TripAdvisor: feedback 95
Tungasuvvingat Inuit (TI) 76

United States of America (USA): children 23; Food and Drug Administration (FDA) 29; insurance 30; services 27–8

Veale, D. 42
violence 78; abuse 75; family 61; safety plans 61

Webber, M.: and Nathan, J. 94
Weber, B. 82
wellness 79; health 9
western culture: woman 40
western psychology 9
Whitaker, R. 29
Wilhelm, S.: and Greenberg, J.L. 40
women: body image 56
World Health Organisation (WHO) 111

Yerushalmi, H. 4, 107–20
Young, I.M. 45
youths 25, 28–9; antipsychotic medication 26; caregivers 29–30; community 81–2; long-term outcome 26–7; onset patterns 25–6; police encounters 53–72